About The Aut

Liz Earle is the health and beauty presenter on ITV's popular *This Morning* programme. Her specialist knowledge and enthusiasm have made her reports compulsive viewing for millions nationwide. A former journalist, Liz has written for many national magazines and newspapers, and was the health and beauty editor of *New Woman* magazine. She is also a regular contributor to radio. Liz has a wealth of inside knowledge about the beauty business and maintains a strong personal interest in complementary medicine.

Beauty is more than skin deep, yet society persists in placing great importance on our appearance. Looking good leads to feeling good, and disfigurement can be a serious disability. For this reason 25 per cent of all royalties received from the sale of this book will be donated to the Laserfair campaign. This is run by the Disfigurement Guidance Centre, Cupar, Fife, a pioneering resource centre that also establishes laser-therapy centres to treat those disfigured from birth or by accidents.

VITAL OILS

Discover the dietary secret of oils and how a few drops each day can improve your health and beauty

Liz Earle

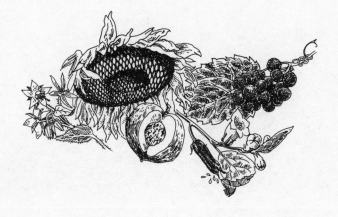

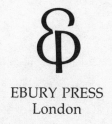

EBURY PRESS
London

In memory of
Sally Tate-Gilder

She walks in beauty, like the night
Of cloudless climes and starry skies;
And all that's best of dark and bright
Meet in her aspect and her eyes:

Byron

Published in 1991 by Ebury Press
an imprint of the Random Century Group
Random Century House
20 Vauxhall Bridge Road
London SW1V 2SA

British Library Cataloguing-in-Publication Data
Earle, Liz
    Vital oils: Discover the dietary secret of oils
    and how a few drops each day
    can improve your health and beauty. – (Ebury Press)
    I. Title   II. Series
    612.3

    ISBN 0-09-174974-3

        Front cover design by Sue Sharples

Typeset in Palatino by ⧘Tek Art Limited, Croydon, Surrey
Printed and bound in Great Britain by Mackays of Chatham Plc

Contents

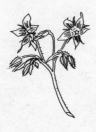

Acknowledgments

This book is the realisation of a dream, and there are many people who deserve heartfelt thanks for helping me turn an ambition into reality. Foremost, I should like to thank Beverley Benson for her encouragement. I have been fortunate enough to work with many of the leading lights of the 'oil field' and must express my deep gratitude to all the research scientists and other health-care professionals who painstakingly explained their complicated subjects to me in layman's language. These include Tom Hardman, Caroline Wheeler, Willem vas Dias, Professor Colin Ratledge, Dr Roger Leysen, Hilary Robinson, Dr Stephan Wright, Jan Kusmerik, Andrew Jedwell, Eoin Mullarney, Marie Erdmann, Val Holmes, Signor Juan Vincente Gomez Moya, Dr David Atherton and Penny Upritchard of the Hospital For Sick Children, Great Ormond Street. Also Nigel Earle, Sarah Collins, Stephanie Goff, Karen Berman, Janis Raven, Mark Constantine, Sue Butler and the Fish Foundation in Tiverton, Devon.

A very special thank-you to Dr Ray Rice for checking my every word on a complicated subject that he *still* knows far more about than I do. Also to food writer and nutritionist Anne Gains for helping me with the *Vital Oils Beauty Diet* and for devising the delicious, oil-enriched recipes. My knowledge of aromatherapy was greatly broadened by many aromatherapists and I am especially grateful to the lovely Geraldine Howard for information on the use of linseed poultices and for her general enthusiasm. Her magical hands also helped to keep tension at bay during lengthy sessions at the word processor.

Last, but not least, my thanks to all those who supported me while writing this book. Especially my producer, Kay Gordon and the editor of *This Morning*, Liam Hamilton. To my mother, Ann Bawtree, Diana Rattan and Laura Hill who lovingly looked after my new-born daughter Lily – and to Lily herself for (mostly) sleeping through the night. Finally, I thank my husband Patrick, whose ceaseless support and encouragement made all the difference in the world.

Introduction

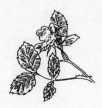

Natural oils have been described as the life-force of a plant and many are famed for their healing properties. Vegetable oils from nuts and seeds have played an important part in many ancient cultures, both as powerful medicines and effective beauty treatments. Plant oils are an amazingly concentrated source of the nutrients needed for life. These include vitamins, minerals and most important of all, a group of substances called essential fatty acids. These nutrients are required by every living cell in our body to function properly and a lack of these essential fatty acids can contribute to many of the ailments associated with modern life, such as heart disease, cancer and stress. Low levels of essential fatty acids in the diet can also lead to many beauty problems including a dry, flaky complexion, weak nails and dull hair. Our eating habits have changed dramatically over the years and many of us now risk a deficiency of these vital oils. In addition, modern food processing has stripped many oils of their naturally healthy assets, robbing us of the important nutrients that ensure good looks as well as health.

This book is about using natural, unprocessed oils to achieve long-lasting health – not simply lack of disease, but also improving your looks, increasing energy levels and generating a positive feeling of well-being. It is also about discovering a renewed vitality and zest for life. Those who have tried the simple, straightforward eating programme have found several positive side-effects, including glowing skin, strong nails and glossy hair. There are so many advantages to be gained from adding these 'vital oils' to our diet and to our skincare regime that they really can provide a healthier, more attractive lifestyle.

This book asks you to increase the amount of oil in your diet, but more importantly it insists on greater care when choosing your oils. Above all, it is the *kind* of oil that is so vitally important. Oils provide energy and nutrients such as vitamins and essential fatty acids – but beware – all oils or fats are not created equal. Some, such as the saturated kind from animal sources, are a positive menace and must be kept to a minimum or avoided altogether. Instead, we should turn to different types of unrefined oils that provide the body with an exotic cocktail of many health-enhancing nutrients. What we eat profoundly affects the way our body performs and by reducing our intake of saturated fats and increasing the amount of other oils in our diet, we can expect to see a vast difference in the way we look and feel. Extensive independent research for the *Vital Oils Beauty Diet* has revealed a huge range of significant health benefits including:

- Increased energy levels
- Clear skin, shiny hair and strong nails
- Greater resistance to heart disease
- Fewer inflammatory disorders such as arthritis
- A stronger immune system.

The Beauty Boosters

The advantages of many oils are not confined to our diet and some of the more exotic oils such as peach kernel and passionflower have properties that benefit our looks as well as our well-being. Oils have been highly prized for their skin-softening properties for thousands of years and were the forerunners to modern skincare. Today, scientists are rediscovering their secrets and have found that some oils significantly improve the condition of our skin, strengthen our nails and give a natural glossy sheen to our hair. These exotic oils are good sources of the oil-soluble vitamins such as A, D and E as well as the essential fatty acids needed by the skin to maintain its tone and elasticity. Many natural oils also contain useful amounts of lecithin which has important water-holding properties. By taking supplements of these oils we can take care of our complexion from the inside-out and even delay the signs of ageing by slowing the formation of fine lines and wrinkles. The essential fatty acids found in oils such as evening primrose and borage oil, for example, help strengthen the delicate membranes surrounding skin cells and make them more able to resist attack from destructive enzymes during the ageing process. These fatty acids also slow signs of ageing by keeping our skin cells functioning in a healthy way for longer. They also help cells resist the attacks from free-radicals that lead to cellular disorganisation and an increased risk of cancer.

Since the earliest civilisations, oils have been an important part of daily life. Their wide-ranging benefits are due to the unique elements that each type of oil contains, and all are vitally important for enhancing our health. Many of the oils mentioned in this book can improve debilitating ailments – but all possess the power to restore vitality and glowing good looks. Make the most of these potent healers by including just a few drops in your life every day and you can expect to feel fitter, less stressed and to enjoy a complexion that positively glows with good health.

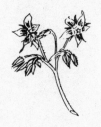

1

Face the Fats

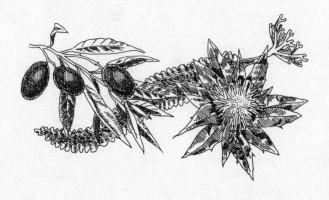

You may think that your oil consumption is confined to the frying pan or to French dressing, but in reality oil is far more prevalent in the form of fats. These can account for up to 40 per cent of our average daily food intake. Fats are simply oils that are solid at room temperature (around 20° C/68° F) and have a similar chemical structure. Getting to grips with the chemical composition of fats and oils is the first step towards achieving better health.

In recent years, no single area of our diet has changed more radically than the type of fats and oils we consume. In an attempt to combat heart disease, lose weight and become generally fitter we have moved away from high-fat foods, increased our intake of low-fat products and in some cases, cut out fatty foods altogether. The next time you are in the supermarket cast your eyes over the huge array of low-cholesterol and fat-free products and you will soon realise the amazing culinary revolution that has taken place on the shelves. The terminology is bewildering too, with words like polyunsaturated and hydrogenated littered across the labels. The wording high in polyunsaturates leads us to believe that a product will somehow be good for us – but is this really true? And how many truly understand the new terminology and its implications for our health? I for one will admit to having been totally baffled by the bewildering array of biochemical labelling, which is why the beginning of this book explores – and in some cases explodes – some of the myths perpetrated by the food industry. What must be remembered is the wide range of health benefits that oils bring – and that the trend towards a fat-free diet is a big mistake in terms of our overall well-being.

A properly balanced diet is one that contains the correct amounts of nutrients needed by the body to function effectively. These include fats, proteins, carbohydrates, vitamins and minerals which should all come, as far as possible, from natural sources. By cutting down on certain fats, such as those in unrefined oils, we run the risk of deficiency in vital substances such as essential fatty acids, which can lead to significant health problems. Essential fatty acids are, as their name implies, essential for good health. When first discovered, essential fatty acids were incorrectly called vitamin F because it was thought that they were vitamins. We now know that they are important substances in their own right, although this collective name is still occassionally mis-used. Essential fatty acids are important for keeping our body tissues in good condition and are vital components of the membranes that surround every living cell. The body cannot make its own supplies of essential fatty acids so we must obtain all we need from the food we eat. However, this does not mean that we should invest in a deep-fat fryer or welcome back the fried breakfast. It is the *type* of oil in our diet – and not the quantity – that is fundamental to maintaining a high level of health and glowing good looks.

Oils as Food

All edible oils and fats come under the biological description of 'lipids' and are largely composed of fatty acids with small amounts of glycerine. They are all 100 per cent fat and have around 125 calories per tablespoonful. Whilst they all look much the same, there is one small chemical characteristic that makes a vast difference to our health.

The fatty acids themselves are large molecules made up of long chains of carbon atoms. Fatty acids vary in structure and may be saturated or unsaturated. In chemical terms, the carbon chains that contain their maximum number of hydrogen atoms are said to be saturated, while those that lack a certain number of hydrogen atoms are said to be unsaturated. Just as the composition of each oil differs from one kind to another – so do the effects they have on the body. Saturated fats are mostly of animal origin such as red meat and dairy produce and are the easiest to identify as they tend to be solid at room temperature (for example lard, butter and cheese). The exceptions to this rule are coconut and palm oils, both from the plant kingdom and both also high in saturates. The reason that we are advised to avoid this type of fat is that a diet high in saturates will increase the "bad" form of cholesterol called low-density lipoprotein (LDL) that encourages deposits in the arteries and raises the risk of heart attacks and thrombosis. Saturated fats are also bad news because they block the health-enhancing properties of other, more beneficial types of lipids.

There are two types of unsaturated fats – poly- and monounsaturated – most of which are vegetable in origin. Fish also contain significant levels of polyunsaturates, although these have a slightly different structure to those from vegetable sources. Chemically speaking, the polyunsaturated kind has fewest hydrogen atoms linked to its chain of carbon molecules. Polyunsaturated fats, such as sunflower or safflower oil, reduce the levels of harmful LDL in the bloodstream and are often promoted in low-fat diets. However, recent medical evidence suggests that polyunsaturated fats have the unwanted side-effect of reducing levels of the beneficial type of cholesterol called high-density lipoprotein (HDL), whose function is to prevent cholesterol deposits from settling in our arteries. The normal ratio of HDL to LDL is thought to be 1:5, which means that the HDL has to work hard to carry the cholesterol away from the cells and back to the liver, where it is converted into bile acid prior to excretion. However, an excess of polyunsaturates may disrupt the delicate balance between the lipoproteins, tipping it in favour of the less desirable LDLs. This news casts a shadow over the health-giving claims made by the makers of polyunsaturated spreads and cooking oils, and has led to heated debates between the food industry and some medics. Perhaps more importantly though, many polyunsaturated products are highly processed by the time they reach our shopping trolley and this refining destroys many of their benefits.

The Cholesterol Connection

Polyunsaturated oils are a relatively new discovery, yet in the last decade alone our consumption has increased three-fold. While this is good news for the makers of highly refined margarine and cooking oils, it is less encouraging for our health. So how did the polyunsaturates become so popular? The story of their success relates to cholesterol, the waxy substance that has been closely linked with heart disease. Cholesterol is used in the body as a component of the membranes surrounding every living cell. Its function is to ensure that the fats we need to transport can be moved around in the largely water-based fluids such as blood and lymph. Cholesterol also helps keep our nerve fibres in good condition and is needed for the manufacture of hormones. Because cholesterol is important to us biologically, the body is capable of making its own supplies. This takes place in the liver, and the less cholesterol we eat, the harder our liver works to replace it. So no matter what we spread on our toast, it is impossible to cut cholesterol out of our lives altogether. Not only is it impossible to cut out cholesterol, it would be highly unwise as it is an essential biochemical that the body can not do without. However, the food industry has latched on to the idea that cholesterol is the principle culprit when it comes to heart disease.

While cholesterol has received an extremely bad press there is no disputing that it can clog up our arteries, like limescale furring up pipework. But the problem cholesterol causes is not entirely due to the substance itself. The unwanted build-up of cholesterol is simply a symptom of the body not being able to process its blood fats correctly, and this comes down to the type of oils in our diet. The only way to ensure that we have a healthy balance of blood fats and encourage the formation of high-density lipoprotein (HDL) is to not only cut down on our saturated fats but also to limit the use of highly refined fats (such as low-fat spreads) and heat-treated cooking oils. These over-processed products are not as nutritious and should be replaced with healthier alternatives. The good news is that there are many alternatives readily available to us and I call these our *vital oils*. In their raw, natural and unrefined state, plant oils such as olive, almond and sesame seed are bursting with health benefits. These oils are all monounsaturated and have the ability to regulate our delicate balance of lipoproteins. By using these oils we're able to prevent an excessive amount of LDL from forming, while maintaining or even increasing levels of the beneficial HDL. In addition, fish oil supplements have also been found to be extremely useful in preventing excessive LDL levels in the bloodstream.

Cooking Oils

Saturated	Polyunsaturated	Monounsaturated
coconut	safflower	olive
palm	sunflower	almond
butter	walnut	hazelnut
lard	grapeseed	avocado
margarine	soya bean	groundnut (peanut)
	pumpkin	pistachio
	corn	sesame
	rapeseed	

Unrefined Tastes

You will notice that in referring to the type of oils we should be eating I use the all-important words natural and unrefined. This is because it is not only the type of oil that matters, the way they are processed is crucial too. The chemical makeup of every oil that ends up in a bottle on the supermarket shelf depends on the way it is refined. In the good old days, oils were extracted by cold-pressing methods involving the coarse grinding of nuts and seeds before pressing to release the oil. This was (and still is) a time-consuming and costly exercise which is also wasteful as it leaves much of the oil behind. It takes about 5 kilos (11 lb) of olives to make just 1 litre (1¾ pints) of cold-pressed olive oil, usually extracted from hard, unripe olives. In the 19th century, a screw-press method of extraction was invented which was more effective as it applied greater mechanical pressure to release the oils. Later still it was discovered that if the oil-laden nuts or seeds were heated up to a temperature of 100°C (212°F) before pressing, even more oil would be released. Although heated pressing is still used today to some extent, there are definite nutritional drawbacks. When polyunsaturated fatty acids are heated it triggers the process known as oxidation, which means the fatty acid molecules combine with oxygen molecules at a much faster rate than normal. It is this oxidation that destroys vital nutrients within oils, such as vitamin E and the essential fatty acids – which, as their name suggests – are essential for achieving good health.

The main method of oil extraction employed by cooking-oil manufacturers today is equally unappealing. Solvent extraction uses petroleum derivatives to dissolve the oils and make the whole extraction process faster and more effective. The principal solvent used is hexane, a major component of petrol, which evaporates at relatively low temperatures. Solvent extraction and oil refining is a lengthy process and these are the stages of its treatment:

- Mechanical pressing of seeds at intense pressure and high temperatures up to 200°C (400°F).
- Residual grounds cooked and pressed again.
- Remaining oilcake mixed with solvent (such as petrol-based hexane). The solvent oil mixture is drained away from the residual cake and then heated to 150°C (300°F) and hexane removed by vacuum distillation.
- Resulting blend is dark and evil-smelling. It is degummed by re-heating and spraying with hot water. This removes all valuable phospholipids, including lecithin.
- Any remaining free fatty acids are destroyed by alkali refining using caustic soda.
- Natural pigments are removed by bleaching. This involves mixing the oil with earths treated with acid to make them more absorbent. The pigments cling on to the earths and are filtered out.

- Finally the oil's natural flavours and aromas are removed by deodorisation. The oil is heated to 250°C (480°F) and pressurised steam is blown through to collect these compounds which accumulate on the surface. This also removes all traces of vitamin E.

By contrast, unrefined oils involve the single mechanical pressing of seeds at temperatures usually below 80°C (175°F). The oil is then filtered and bottled.

The only method of extraction that preserves the original goodness of an oil is cold-pressing. Any chef will also tell you that cold-pressed oils are the tastiest, because the refining drives away the volatile flavour compounds that give certain oils their unique flavour. Unfortunately, cold-pressed oils are the the most inefficient to produce and are also the most expensive, which explains why virgin olive oil made from the first pressing of olives can cost more than champagne!

Cooking Oils

The problems that occur when an oil is heated also mean that we must choose our methods of cooking very carefully. Heating an oil to a high temperature, for instance in a chip pan, destroys all the healthy properties we want to preserve. When oil is heated above 100°C (212°F) it not only wipes out important nutrients, but also generates free-radicals. These destructive molecular fragments have been implicated in all kinds of health scares, from heart disease to cancer and even premature ageing. Free-radicals are formed when the double bonds in the chemical structure of unsaturated fatty acids are attacked by oxygen molecules. This generates hydro-peroxides, highly unstable molecules capable of causing multiple cell damage throughout the body. It is this cell damage that is thought to be a precursor to cancer and encourage premature skin and body ageing. However, nature has an innate sense of balance and many vegetable oils are naturally enriched with vitamin E, a nutrient renowned for its extraordinary health-giving properties. Most important of these is its ability to seek out and neutralise free-radicals, thereby minimising the amount of internal cell damage. However, as vitamin E is also destroyed in the heating process, using oils at high temperatures not only creates free-radicals but also destroys the very weapons needed to combat them. Peanut oil, for example, is a rich source of vitamin E, but frying at high temperatures will reduce its vitamin E levels by one-third. Amongst the least stable oils for cooking are sunflower, safflower, soya bean and rapeseed, all of which produce high levels of free-radicals when heated. If you really *must* fry the occasional meal choose olive oil as it is less prone to the whole process of oxidation. But only use the oil once and never re-heat.

Off the Shelf

As the benefits of cold-pressed oils become more widely known, so they become increasingly available, but unfortunately there is a sting in the tale. As yet there is no legislation to control the exact labelling of oils, and an oil may state that it has been cold-pressed even if it has subsequently been subjected to heat-treating or further refined after the cold pressing. In addition, the crushing process may have been carried out with great force or speed which generates its own heat, technically making the oil warm pressed. Some enlightened oil producers have recognised this difficulty and describe their products as unrefined, which is probably the most accurate description. Other manufacturers are not so up-front, making it extremely difficult for us to know exactly what is in the bottle. However, there are a few ground rules that can help us decide what to buy:

- Choose oils that are naturally darker in colour and have a nutty smell. These qualities indicate that an oil has not been bleached or deodorised.
- Stick to the single oils instead of those that state they are a blend of several different varieties. With a pure oil, at least you know what type you're getting.
- Choose oils that have been packaged to protect them from rancidity caused by exposure to the light. Look for dark-coloured glass bottles or metal containers.
- Check the best-before date. Unrefined oils should keep for nine months due to their natural antioxidants.

- Every time you take the top off an oil bottle, the contents come under attack from oxygen molecules, so choose smaller bottles and replace more frequently instead of buying in bulk.

Once purchased, store the oils in a cool, dark place away from sunlight. Some natural clouding may occur (particularly in cold weather), and is a welcome sign that the oil has not been refined or excessively filtered. The fridge is one of the best places to keep oil and a few days of cold-storage will tell you more about the oil too. If it appears cloudy or develops sediment do not panic, as refrigeration encourages the saturated portion of the oil to sink to the bottom. Those keen to reduce their saturated fatty acid levels can simply leave this inch or so behind in the bottle. Unrefined vegetable oils that still retain their nutrients will quickly lose them if stored at room temperature. Safflower oil loses more than half its vitamin E after three months and corn oil loses more than one-third after six months. The exception to using cold-storage is olive oil which may solidify at low temperatures. However, olive oil is more resistant to damage by heat and light than polyunsaturated oils and can be safely stored at room temperature.

Supplementary Benefits

While increasing the amount of unrefined cooking oils in our diet will improve overall health and vitality, more acute health problems such as heart disease, arthritis, Pre-Menstrual Syndrome and skin disorders may need specific treatment with oil supplements. Over the years, the medical profession has become increasingly aware of the benefits of oil supplements and a staggering array of capsules now fills the shelves of the chemist and health food shops. But despite the recent focus of attention, taking a daily dose of oil to ward off various ills is nothing new. The Ancient Greeks and Romans used olive oil, for example, to heal scar tissue and sunburn by rubbing it on to the body and scraping it off using a curved wooden blade called a *strigil*. The British Museum has an example of two *strigils* standing in a bronze olive oil pot, thought to have been used by Roman athletes after training sessions. The Romans also favoured olive oil and both Pliny and Hippocrates prescribed it for all kinds of diverse ailments, from insomnia to boils.

Cod liver oil is the biggest selling oil supplement today and it also has a fascinating past. Traditionally taken by the fishermen of Scotland, Iceland and Norway to keep out the cold, the first medical experiments involving cod liver oil were carried out in the 1750s. Samuel Key was a prominent physician at that time and wrote: 'So general has been the use of cod liver oil that we dispense 50 or 60 gallons annually and the good effects of it are so well known among the poorer sort that it is particularly requested by them for almost every lameness. Except bark, opium and mercury, I believe no one medicine in the materia medica is likely to be of better service.' Fortunately cod liver oil has stood the test of time rather better than the rest of his favourite remedies.

Other supplements from the sea to catch the eye of the medical world are the oils extracted from the flesh of fatty fish such as mackerel and herring. These oils contain the fatty acids EPA (eicosapentaenoic acid) and DHA (docosahexaenoic acid) required by the body to make prostaglandins. These hormone-like substances lower the likelihood of heart disease by reducing the risk of blood clots forming in the body. Fish oils are also vitally important for healthy brain cells, proving once and for all the old wives' tale about fish being good for the brain.

Another supplement to arouse particular medical interest is evening primrose oil which contains GLA (gamma linolenic acid) and also influences the production of prostaglandins. Evening primrose oil is one of the most versatile natural healers ever discovered. There is a wealth of scientific evidence to show that it can improve Pre-Menstrual Syndrome, eczema, breast pain and even hyperactivity in children, all of which will be discussed later.

Quackery or Cures?

The alternative health-care industry has more than its fair share of charlatans and quacks, so how can we be sure which oils really are good for our health? After all, the claims are far-reaching and can sound far-fetched. One way to confirm that a substance has been thoroughly researched is to check its medical pedigree. In Great Britain there are three categories of legally recognised medicines. The first is what is known in the trade as a GSL, short for the General Sales List given to pharmacists and chemists. GSLs are licensed by the Department of Health for specific ailments, for example cod liver oil has a product licence for relieving symptoms of arthritis such as joint aches and muscular stiffness. The next step up is the P product – this stands for pharmacy only and so it must be sold by, or in the presence of, a qualified pharmacist. Some fish oil capsules have a Pharmacy Licence and may be dispensed to patients with heart disease to relieve symptoms of hypertriglyceridaemia (raised levels of blood fats). The final category is POM, or Prescription-Only Medicines, and these are available only on prescription from your doctor. Some super-strength evening primrose oil capsules are available on prescription only. Certain brands of evening primrose oil may be prescribed for the treatment of atopic eczema and, more recently, for breast pain.

To qualify for any of these categories the Department of Health must first be satisfied that they are likely to work for the patient. This involves a lengthy process of double-blind clinical trials carried out under the strictest medical supervision. Half those tested are given a placebo or dummy set of capsules (usually filled with liquid paraffin). No one taking part knows whether they are getting the placebo or the real thing, making the point that some patients will improve no matter what they are given! The doctors involved in double-blind trials are also kept in the dark about which participants receive the placebos. This is especially important in cases where the doctor needs to make an impartial judgement on the patient's progress. Clinical trials may take years to complete and it is only when conclusive results have been achieved that a product can be considered for licensing. The fact that so many oil supplements have passed this rigorous procedure is proof of their efficacy.

The Ageing Factor

In Britain we spend a staggering £400 million each year on skincare products for our faces alone and about half this sum is spent on moisturisers. A glance at the cosmetic counters in any department store soon reveals why this amount is so high. Lavishly packaged jars of moisturiser cost small fortunes and their often ridiculously high prices have been known to reach £250. So what is it that prompts us to even consider spending this kind of money on a single pot of face cream? The answer is not only our fear of growing old, but of looking our age. We live in a youth-orientated society, where 15-year-old models stare out at us from magazine covers and the unlined faces of the young advertise anti-wrinkle remedies. Role models such as Raquel Welch, Linda Evans and Joan Collins (all in their fifties) prove that the older woman can be glamorous – provided of course that she doesn't have a line on her face. The jet-set can hide their sagging skin and double chins with a little help from the surgeon's knife, but lesser mortals usually make do with less drastic options. Skincare companies are experts at selling a clever blend of hype and hope in a jar, but do their products really make the skin look younger? That depends on how you define "younger looking". Do you measure the time-lapse in minutes or years? Many of the so-called anti-ageing formulas will slightly improve the appearance of the skin, but they certainly won't turn the clock back very far. The only way to really slow the effects of skin ageing is to tackle the problem from the inside out with a diet rich in nourishing skin foods, and the best source of these is unrefined oils.

To understand the way oils can help us to win the war on wrinkles, it is worth getting to grips with how our skin works and why it ages. The skin is the body's largest organ and weighs between 2.7–3.6 kilos (6–8 lb). Its function is to hold our insides together and protect internal organs from daily hazards such as bacteria and chemical pollutants. Skin is also the body's thermostat, regulating body heat through perspiration while excreting toxins and waste-matter via the pores. It produces its own form of oil called sebum in the sebaceous glands that lie just beneath the surface of the skin. This oil is continually secreted by these glands and its function is to keep the skin moist and supple. Our skin may look static but in fact it is constantly on the move, continually shedding dead skin cells and replacing them with fresh, young ones. These new cells are produced in the lower level of the skin called the dermis and take around 28 days to travel their way up through the different layers of skin to reach the surface. This is why when you try a new skincare regime it takes about a month before you see much difference on your face.

The Skin Nourishers

Many factors influence the way our skin ages. These include hereditary factors that determine the genetic structure of our skin and lifestyle factors such as stress, smoking, alcohol and diet. Of all these variables, our diet is probably the most important and certainly the easiest to change. Our skin needs a rich supply of several vitamins and essential fatty acids to keep it in good condition, all of which are found in oils. Vegetable oils are naturally rich in vitamin E, the most famous skin vitamin. This nutrient is often referred to as the vitality vitamin because of its repairing and regenerating properties within the body.

Vitamin E is an antioxidant, which means that it is able to prevent cell damage from the destructive elements free-radicals. Free-radicals are a normal by-product of the body's metabolism, but in excess they can multiply out of control and damage healthy tissue. Free-radicals also contribute to the ageing process by destroying the collagen and elastin fibres that support the skin. Without this support our skin slackens and loses its youthful firmness. In addition, free-radicals interfere with the formation of fresh, healthy skin cells, making our complexion blotchy and dull. Vitamin E has the ability to neutralise free-radicals as soon as they are formed and will help prevent this trail of damage. Its action as a free-radical scavenger has led to vitamin E being included in an increasing number of skincare products, but the most effective way to use this nutrient is to take it internally.

The value of vitamin E as a nutrient is becoming increasingly known, not just to delay premature ageing but also to prevent a variety of cancers, cataract formation, arthritis and heart disease. Some of the most exciting studies were recently carried out at the Cardiovascular Research and Medical Statistics Units at Edinburgh and the Vitamin Unit at Berne University. These show vitamin E to be valuable in protecting against cardiovascular disorders. Low levels of vitamin E were found to dramatically increase the risk of developing angina (chest pain). One member of the medical team was Professor Michael Oliver, who states that some populations with a high incidence of coronary heart disease may benefit from eating diets rich in natural antioxidants, particularly vitamin E.

Another important vitamin found in oils is vitamin A. This nutrient is used by the body to maintain healthy eyes and vision as well as for repairing skin tissues. Vitamin A controls the rate at which skin cells are shed and replaced by new ones. A shortage of vitamin A leads to a sluggish turnover of cells and a sallow, scaly complexion. Vitamin A deficiencies may also lead to a condition called hyperkeratosis where the fresh, young cells die before they reach the skin's surface, resulting in a dry, flaky complexion. This flaky skin tissue then accumulates with sebum and dirt to form spots and pimples, and can lead to more serious skin disorders such as acne and dandruff.

Vitamin D is the third vital nutrient found in certain oils and is needed for healthy skin and bone development. Vitamin D works with calcium to build bones and teeth, and also affects the quality and tone of skin tissues. This vitamin also promotes healing, and is used in ointments for burns and abrasions.

Unrefined oils are also rich in lecithin. This nutrient occurs in all animal and vegetable cells, and is an important component of cellular membranes. Lecithin also helps make up the myelin sheath that surrounds nerves and also helps our liver metabolise blood fats. The richest sources of lecithin include unrefined soya, peanut and corn oils.

The skin needs more than these nutrients however in order to slow the signs of ageing. Essential fatty acids, such as linoleic acid, are required to build the membranes that surround every skin cell. These fatty acids are also needed to strengthen the protective lipidic barrier that lies beneath the surface of the skin and guards against moisture loss. A diet deficient in essential fatty acids soon shows up on the face and one of the side-effects of a low-fat diet is a dry, devitalised complexion. In the short-term this is not too much of a problem, although parched skin adds years to the face. But starving the skin of its essential fatty acids for long periods of time leads to serious skin problems and premature ageing. In addition, a lack of linoleic acid reduces the strength of the skin's supporting collagen fibres, may slow wound healing and can even trigger hair loss. Polyunsaturated vegetable oils are the richest sources of linoleic acid, the parent of other essential fatty acids such as gamma linolenic acid (GLA). However, many of these polyunsaturates are heated to high temperatures during their refining and this dramatically alters their chemical structure. We know that once a polyunsaturated oil has been heated above 100°C (212°F) it increases the risk of peroxidation, a process that encourages free-radical cell damage. In addition, the polyunsaturates that end up in most margarines and low-fat spreads have gone through a process of hydrogenation which reduces essential fatty acids. Hydrogenation also converts some of the polyun-saturates into trans-fatty-acids which behave in a similar way to saturated fats in the body. Researchers in Holland have found that eating hydrogenated margarine alters the LDL:HDL ratio in the bloodstream, and may increase the risk of heart disease. So, if you see the words 'hydro-genated vegetable oil' on the label, read it as 'saturated fat' and think carefully before buying. The commercial fats used in food processing also contain up to 50 per cent hydrogenated fat, yet another reason why highly refined foods are to be avoided. The only way to ensure we receive our vital supplies of essential fatty acids and vitamins is to opt for the unrefined vegetable oils that still retain their precious health-giving properties.

2
The Healing Oils

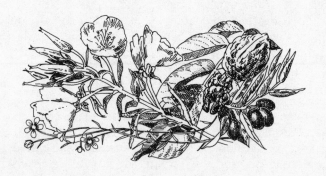

Edible oils are naturally enriched with nutrients that improve the way we look and feel. Some, such as olive oil, are easily incorporated into our daily diet, while others, such as the fish oils, avocado and evening primrose oil, come in capsule form and can be swallowed as supplements. Many possess the power to relieve acute ailments such as heart disease and atopic eczema, but all have the ability to improve energy levels and vitality. Plant oils have been used as natural healers for thousands of years and many can be traced back to the Ancient Greeks and Egyptians. Today, scientists are able to analyse their unique chemical structures and can identify the active ingredients in each oil. And although most plant oils look the same, once inside the body they behave in very different ways. This chapter details the edible oils most readily available to us.

Almond Oil (Prunus amygdalus)

The History

The almond tree is a native of the Middle East and now flourishes in the warm, sunny climates of the Mediterranean and California. It was first brought to Britain by the Romans and can be traced back to biblical times. The Rod of Aaron mentioned in the Bible is thought to have been a branch from the almond tree and twigs of almond blossom are still carried in some Jewish festivals. There are two varieties of tree, the sweet almond (*dulcis*) and bitter almond (*amara*), and both varieties flower in January with a profusion of frothy white blossom. The almonds form on short branches and are protected by a tough outer husk that resembles a greengage. Because of this fleshy covering almonds belong to the same fruit family as peaches and apricots, although their pulp is nowhere near as tasty. When the almonds are harvested the outer case splits open to reveal the nut inside. Cold-pressing the kernels yields up to half their weight in oil.

The Science

The description almond oil almost invariably refers to sweet almond oil as this is the variety most widely used. Bitter almond oil should be treated with caution as it contains traces of amygdalin which can be hydrolised or distilled to produce deadly hydrocyanic acid (cyanide). Almond oil is highly nutritious, being a good source of nutrients, such as trace minerals and the essential polyunsaturate linolenic acid. It is also a useful source of linoleic acid. In its raw state immediately after extraction, almond oil is a pale yellow colour. However, the oil usually undergoes an extensive bleaching and refining process that renders it completely colourless and also robs it of its nutritional value. The pharmaceutical industry is a major buyer of almond oil and it is used as a base for ointments as well as in mild laxatives.

Health Benefits

Almond oil is a good source of monounsaturated fatty acids and its most recent role is in the prevention of heart disease. Researchers in America have discovered almond oil to be twice as effective as the better-known olive oil in reducing the build-up of cholesterol. Clinical trials published in the American *Journal of Clinical Nutrition* report that after just four weeks on an almond-based diet, the participants' cholesterol levels dropped by an average of 11 per cent. Other control groups taking part in the study included those on an olive-based diet, whose cholesterol levels dropped by an average of 5 per cent, and those on a saturated fat diet high in butter and cheese, whose cholesterol levels not surprisingly increased. Those on the almond diet ate natural almonds and ground almonds and were only allowed to use almond oil for cooking. As a result of this data, the Almond Board of California is now urging Americans to use almonds at every culinary opportunity, from sprinkling ground almonds on to yogurt or waffles for breakfast to extending chicken casseroles with these nutritious nuts. Almond oil could also be used in recipes instead of other monounsaturated oils such as olive oil, but would prove far too expensive.

Borage Oil (Borago officinalis)

The History

The Romans called borage the herb of gladness and used an infusion from its leaves to treat depression. Originally from Aleppo in Syria, borage is now grown all over Europe. It is easily recognisable in the herb bed by its bright blue flowers and rough greyish green leaves. Although borage is not especially aromatic it attracts bees in the garden and has the nickname 'beebread'. Its flavour is similar to that of cucumber and it is a traditional addition to cold drinks in the summer. During the Middle Ages borage was a popular anti-inflammatory agent and was also used to treat rheumatism and heart disease. The English herbalist Nicholas Culpeper was ahead of his time when he described borage seeds as being useful for increasing the milk in women's breasts, as borage has only recently been identified as one of the richest sources of GLA, the essential fatty acid naturally present in breast milk. Having been relegated over the years to little more than a garnish for glasses of fruit punch, the borage plant is now staging a dramatic come-back.

The Science

As a result of the research into the medicinal effects of evening primrose oil and its essential fatty acids, scientists began to search for other natural sources of GLA. But what could be better than the evening primrose? The answer is borage, a common British herb whose seeds contain over twice as much GLA as evening primrose oil. In fact, borage seeds consist of a staggering 25 per cent pure GLA, which means that it is more than twice as concentrated as evening primrose oil. The good news for consumers is that because it contains twice as much GLA, we only need half as much of it to achieve the same effect. This means swallowing fewer capsules which should, in theory, cost us less. However, borage has yet to capture the imagination of the nation in the same way that evening primrose oil has done (or is simply not as profitable for the producers), and has yet to become as widely available. However, it can only be a matter of time before the extraordinary benefits of this plant oil are fully acknowledged.

Cod Liver Oil

The History

Physicians used cod liver oil to treat rheumatism and gout as long ago as the 18th century, when it was naively thought that the oil benefited the body by lubricating our joints. Some of the first medical experiments involving cod liver oil were carried out by Dr Samuel Kay in 1752 at Manchester Infirmary. He used it to treat bone disorders and rheumatic pain, and it later became widely used for diseases related to malnutrition, such as rickets. The medical profession accepted that cod liver oil worked and was a useful cure, but no-one knew just *how* it worked.

Nowadays we know that its health benefits come from the fat-soluble vitamins A and D, together with high levels of polyunsaturated fatty acids.

Cod liver oil does literally come from the liver of the cod, most of which are caught in the North Atlantic waters around Iceland and Norway. Deep-sea trawling is a laborious business and involves sinking nets 190 fathoms deep over an area several miles long. The nets are hauled in 2–3 hours after dropping and the fish swim up to the top of the net where their escape is blocked with a knot. This is called the cod end, hence the trawlermen's expression 'it all comes out of a cod end'. The cod has an unusually large liver and it can take just 10 livers to produce one gallon of cod liver oil. In the old days, the fish was landed and cleaned on the quayside and the livers tossed into large oak barrels, where they were left to rot. After a period of days or even weeks, the oil would ooze out from the liver cells as they disintegrated – and we can only imagine the stench. As the oil floated up to the top of the barrel it was skimmed off and strained, ready for bottling. The oil produced in this way was a dark, evil-smelling brew and was sold mainly to the tanning industry for softening leather hides. It was a small, but lucrative sideline for the trawlermen, who treated the proceeds as pin-money. This changed in the mid-1850s when cod liver oil was found to be an effective cure for rickets. This debilitating childhood bone disease causes bow-legs and tragic malformations of the joints and is due to a lack of vitamin D. During the Industrial Revolution rickets was common amongst the children of the workhouses, who spent much of their undernourished lives working in appalling factory conditions. The plight of these children was powerfully portrayed by Charles Dickens, and there is no doubt that Tiny Tim would have benefited from a daily dose of cod liver oil.

When doctors discovered that cod liver oil could prevent and even cure rickets, the demand soared. It became clear that simply leaving the cod livers in barrels to rot was an inefficient means of production. So the steam extraction process was developed which involved boiling up the livers in huge vats and siphoning off the oil. These vats were fitted into the cargo holds of the trawlers and to compensate for the extra workload the fishermen were paid liver money. The production of cod liver oil became big business – and caused intense competition amongst the fishing fleets. This rivalry finally ended for one group in the 1930s when several fleet owners in Hull got together and decided that their time would be better spent working with, and not against, one other. They formed the British Cod Liver Oil Producers Ltd (later re-named Seven Seas), a co-operative that marketed the oil and passed the proceeds back to the men on the boats.

At about this time vitamin D was identified for the first time and found to be present in cod liver oil, and at last doctors began to understand one of the reasons why the supplement is so valuable. Later, when food rationing was in force during and after the Second World War, the Ministry of Food organised free distribution of cod liver oil to all children under five, and to pregnant and breast-feeding women, to prevent malnutrition. After the war, the Welfare Foods Scheme decided that this should continue as, despite the rigours of rationing, Britain's war babies were the healthiest the nation had ever seen.

Although we think of rickets as a disease from the past, some races in Britain remain at risk even now. These include the large Asian communities who have settled in Glasgow, Birmingham, Manchester and Leeds. In addition to obtaining vitamin D from our diet, we also synthesise it through our skin when it is exposed to sunlight. Although the feeble British sunshine suits the fair-skinned British, darker skinned races have more difficulty absorbing sufficient to make vitamin D. This is a particular problem for the Asian communities as they tend to cover themselves up when outdoors. The result can be a serious vitamin D deficiency, and this has led to a worrying resurgence of rickets amongst Asian children. The Department of Health has launched a campaign to make the Asian community more aware of the risks to their children and is once again advocating the use of cod liver oil.

Since its discovery, many more health benefits from cod liver oil have been identified, and what was once the trawlerman's sideline now rivals the fishing catch itself in terms of importance.

The Science

The main nutrients found in cod liver oil are vitamins A and D. Both vitamins are stored in the fat cells of the liver and are said to be fat-soluble. Vitamin D regulates growth and also improves the tensile strength of teeth and bones by controlling calcium absorption. While the body can manufacture some of its own supplies through the skin, this amount can need supplementing. The richest sources of vitamin D are (in order) halibut liver oil, cod liver oil, herring, mackerel, salmon and sardines. Vitamin A is an important nutrient for healthy eyes, skin and hair and for building our resistance to respiratory infections. Because the vitamins in cod liver oil are retained by the body and stored in the liver, it is important not to take them in vast quantities which could be potentially hazardous. The recommended daily dose of most cod liver oil supplements is 10 ml (two teaspoonfuls), although some health practitioners suggest increasing this to 20 ml (one tablespoonful).

Health Benefits

Cod liver oil is one of only a handful of dietary supplements to be granted a medical licence. In this case it is for relieving the pain caused by aching joints and muscles. But to assume that the oil works by simply lubricating the joints is somewhat of an over-simplification. Cod liver oil contains a group of polyunsaturated essential fatty acids called Omega-3. These differ in subtle but very important ways from the polyunsaturated essential fatty acids found in vegetable oils which are called Omega-6. The Omega-3 essential fatty acids come from linolenic acid and are used by the body for the production of prostaglandins (as with evening primrose oil) and also leukotrienes. These are similar to prostaglandins in that they control functions such as blood pressure and the digestion, but they also regulate inflammatory disorders. The level of leukotrienes in the body must be carefully balanced. Too many leukotrienes can result in them instructing cells to begin harmful disease processes such as blood clots and inflammation. Cod liver oil is able to regulate the leukotrienes, making it a very useful supplement in the battle against inflammatory disorders such as arthritis.

One of the best-known cod liver oil enthusiasts of this century was American laboratory technician Dale Alexander, otherwise known as the Cod Father. His passion for this amber nectar stemmed from the fact that it cured his mother's painful arthritis, and *Arthritis and Common Sense* was the first of five books he wrote on the subject. The Cod Father advocated a tablespoonful of cod liver oil a day mixed with milk to disguise what he called its three flavours 'ucky, yucky and bloody awful'. The first scientific paper published on cod liver oil and arthritis appeared in a 1959 edition of *The Journal of the National Medicine Association*. This described a study where 98 patients were given 20 ml of cod liver oil mixed with milk or orange juice, taken on an empty stomach. A 92 per cent success rate in relieving pain and swelling was recorded, with many patients also noticing improved hair, skin and nail condition. It was also noted at the time that part of the success of the oil may have been due to taking it on an empty stomach. Subsequent double-blind clinical trials carried out at Albany Medical College in New York during the 1980s also confirm cod liver oil to be effective for relieving morning stiffness and tender joints. It has also been used with success to treat inflammatory skin conditions.

Other Fish Oils

Of course, there is far more to fish than cod liver oil, and health benefits can be found in every form of fish – from a sardine sandwich to the latest fish oil capsules. We grow up to believe that fish is good for us, yet few of us know exactly why. Amidst the mass of generally accepted folklore lies the theory that fish feeds the heart and brain and there is increasing scientific evidence to support this belief. Fish oils thin the blood so reducing the risk of blood clotting. They have also been linked to increased mental energy and play a vital role in brain development. Fish oils are rich in the fatty acid DHA, and this is the principle polyunsaturate found in the thinking part of the brain. Studies involving rats have found that if they are raised without DHA in their diet, their offspring are less mentally alert. DHA is vitally important for human intelligence too. And we know there is an enormous surge in DHA levels in the brain of an unborn child during the last three months of pregnancy. Some scientists suggest that babies born prematurely may be at risk due to a DHA deficiency and baby food manufacturers are being urged to consider adding DHA to feeds for premature babies. Over the last decade, fish oils have been subjected to close medical scrutiny since the discovery that they are able to alter our balance of blood fats. This is another important attribute of the polyunsaturated essential fatty acid group, Omega-3.

The only organisms to manufacture their own plentiful supplies of Omega-3 EFAs are the single-cell plankton that live in the depths of the ocean. Fish are rich in these essential fatty acids simply because plankton is their main source of food and the Omega-3 EFAs are stored in their fat tissues. This is why oily fish such as herring and mackerel are a far better source of these than white fish such as haddock or plaice. Further up the food chain, seals and whales also have high levels of Omega-3 EFAs as their diet consists entirely of fish. And the Eskimos, who live largely on whale and seal blubber, are one of the few populations with a diet that is naturally enriched with these essential fatty acids.

Health Benefits

The Eskimos in Greenland came under observation when researchers noticed that as a race they rarely suffer heart disease and have no incidence of diabetes. This is despite the fact that seal and whale blubber are both high in cholesterol, which has been linked to heart disease. However, if the Eskimos moved to Canada and adopted the same diet as the Canadians, their incidence of heart disease went up to match that of the Canadians. Clearly something in their homeland was influencing the Eskimos' health, and attention focused on the Eskimo diet which is very rich in Omega-3s.

The Omega-3 polyunsaturates were found to have the extraordinary ability of reducing a group of blood fats called triglycerides. While the Eskimos were found to have similar cholesterol levels to us, their triglyceride levels are only about a quarter compared to those of Westerners. Triglycerides are fat molecules consisting of three fatty acids (hence the name tri-glyceride). High levels of triglycerides in the bloodstream can hinder the body's natural ability to break down clots. This can lead to thrombosis, caused when a clot forms within a blood vessel and blocks the blood supply to important areas of the body such as the heart or brain. Thrombosis can rapidly result in a heart attack or stroke and is the principal cause of death for people in Britain over the age of 45. So important was the discovery of the link between the Omega-3s and heart disease that in 1982 Professor J. R. Vane was awarded the Nobel Prize for medicine for his work on the subject.

Since then, further inroads have been made into how fish oils affect the structure of our blood. We know they dramatically reduce triglyceride levels but they also increase the elasticity of red blood cells. These cells need to be especially pliable in order to flow freely down the finest capillaries in the body, which are often less than 1 mm thick. Red blood cells can be as much as three times the diameter of these tiny blood vessels, but are still able to squeeze through. If the red blood cells loose their elasticity they are unable to reach the surface of the skin, the brain or the heart and blood supplies to these vital organs dwindle. This can result in life-threatening problems such as a heart attack.

Almost one third of us will die from heart disease and it is Britain's biggest killer of both men and women. However this appallingly high figure can be reduced and there is no reason why any of us should become just another statistic. Checking your level of blood fats is one simple way of detecting if you are at risk. Over half the population of America have their blood fats analysed at some time by a simple blood test, yet in this country the figure is a pathetic 5 per cent. Pin-prick blood tests are available at many health food shops and chemists, or your GP will be able to arrange one for you. Another simple, if less scientific, way of assessing cholesterol levels is to gaze into your eyes. A raised cholesterol level often shows up as a milky white ring surrounding the iris or coloured portion of the eye. Common amongst the elderly, this cholesterol ring can show up in those as young as 25.

Reducing the amount of harmful triglycerides means eating more fish oil. In the past, fish was plentiful and cheap and was a major part of the average Briton's diet. In the 18th century masters were even taken to task for making their apprentices eat salmon every day. But one thing the nation did not suffer from was heart disease. Nowadays, we eat far less fish and the the type we do eat such as cod, haddock and plaice, contains the least amount of oil. In addition, many of our fish are reared in farms and fed on soya meal or grain which lack the essential fatty acids plankton contains. Those who can not stand the thought of eating oily fish such as mackerel or herring every day can supplement their diet with a fish oil capsule. Look for the wording pure fish oil on the package which means that the oil has not been chemically processed and the basic construction of the Omega-3s has been preserved.

> *Fish Rich in Omega-3 EFAs (in order)*
> Mackerel
> Herrings
> Sardines
> Bluefin Tuna
> Lake Trout
> Salmon
> Anchovies
> Sprats
> Mullet
> Halibut
> Bass
> Rainbow Trout
> Carp
> Squid

NB: Tuna should be bought fresh and not tinned as the fish oil is drained off and replaced with refined vegetable oils.

Evening Primrose Oil (Oenothera biennis)

The History

The evening primrose is a tall, spiky but elegant plant that only blooms in the evening, hence its common name. In reality it is not a primrose at all, but a spindly wild flower more closely related to the garden flower godetia, and also the rosebay willow herb. Its origins can be traced back 70,000 years to its first appearance in Central America and Mexico. Although evening primroses often grow alongside rivers and streams, these vivid yellow flowers can also be found flourishing in the desert. North American Indian medicine-men were the first to recognise its potential as a healer and brewed the seed pods to make an infusion for healing wounds. They also made poultices from the leaves to soothe aches and sprains and used the juice from its roots as a cough mixture. Later adopted by herbalists, its leaves were used to make mild disinfectants, sedatives and diuretics. The Romans also respected its powers and early translations from Pliny state 'it is an herbe good as wine to make the heart merrie. Of such virtue is this herbe that if it be given to drink to the wildest beast that is, it will tame the same and make it gentle.' In 1650, the English herbalist Nicholas Culpeper also records his use of the evening primrose saying 'it opens obstructions of the liver and spleen, provokes urine, is good for the dropsy if infused in common drink.' Dropsy is the old-fashioned word for oedema, or swelling, and is not a disease in itself but a sign of kidney or heart failure.

Traditionally called the King's Cure-All, over a thousand different types of evening primrose plant have now been identified worldwide. According to geologists, the evening primrose colonised North America at least four times – narrowly escaping extinction during successive ice-ages. It was officially brought to Britain by the English naturalist John Tradescant the younger in the late 17th century. He called it the Yellow Herb of Virginia and it was subsequently re-named the tree primrose. Later, towards the end of the 18th century, the newly established trade routes between North America and Europe brought many more of the seeds to Britain. These seeds were stowaways aboard the many merchant ships, which were loaded with extra ballast for stability in the form of stones, sand and soil. The soil contained evening primrose seeds which germinated and colonised the coastline close to where the ballast was eventually discarded. Even today I have spotted clumps of evening primroses around Liverpool on my weekly travels to Granada Television.

The Science

In addition to its impressive history the evening primrose continues to gather accolades, although medical attention now focuses solely on the oil-bearing seeds of this remarkable plant. The seeds were first analysed in 1919 and found to be rich in fatty acids, including one in particular, identified for the first time as gamma linolenic acid (GLA). Its composition was found to be about 90 per cent unsaturated fatty acids, of which 9 per cent is GLA. At about this time the whole family of fatty acids called essential fatty acids (EFAs) were being identified and their importance in our diet recognised. We now know that these nutrients are needed to maintain healthy body tissues and are also important components of the membranes surrounding every living cell.

The body has difficulty making sufficient amounts of GLA, so we need to obtain extra supplies from the foods we eat. Good sources include vegetables (especially the green, leafy kind), vegetable oils, seeds and pulses. These foods all contain small amounts of linoleic acid which the body then converts to GLA. However, in many people this vital process is blocked by a build-up of saturated fats or highly processed cooking oils or margarine. Poor nutrition may also be a factor, as the conversion process also requires the presence of other nutrients such as vitamin B6, zinc and magnesium. Health problems such as diabetes, viral infections and hormone changes, including pregnancy and the menopause, will also block much of the conversion. Factors such as old age, alcohol and smoking also hinder the process. However, essential fatty acids are vital for good health so it is very important that the body either converts sufficient supplies or receives supplements from a enriched source such as evening primrose oil. To emphasise their importance, the World Health Organisation advises that essential fatty acids should make up at least 3 per cent of our total calorific intake and that this should increase to 5–6 per cent for children and breast-feeding women. Interestingly, one of the few sources of gamma linolenic acid itself is human breast milk, a substance renowned for its nourishment and ability to protect the immune system.

The gamma linolenic acid found in evening primrose oil is biologically important as it effects much of the enzyme activity in our body. Every process that takes place within us is triggered by the action of various enzymes, including the production of prostaglandins. These are hormone-like substances that regulate bodily functions including blood pressure, digestion and inflammation. They were discovered in the 1930s by a Swedish scientist called U. S. von Euler, who identified a substance in the prostate gland and so named it prostaglandin. Since then, approximately 36 different prostaglandins have been identified and occur in every cell in the body. Prostaglandins regulate the movement of material between individual cells, control cell-to-cell communication and the transmission of signals between nerve cells. Although biochemists have yet to pin-point exactly how all prostaglandins work at a molecular level, these hormone-like substances seem to exercise control over just about anything and everything in the body. Unlike hormones though, prostaglandins are not secreted from glands in the body and then transported to where they are needed. Instead, we are able to produce them on the spot in response to a stimulus anywhere in the body. Also unlike hormones, prostaglandins live for only a few seconds before being broken down, which is why we need a steady supply of GLA to ensure our prostaglandin levels remain stable. Their action as regulators and internal messengers means they have a dramatic effect on our overall health and each year literally thousands of medical research papers are recorded involving prostaglandin activity.

Health Benefits

On a personal note, my first encounter with evening primrose oil was five years ago during a particularly bad attack of eczema. I have had a lifetime's experience of this skin disorder and would watch it flare up with depressing regularity during periods of stress or overwork. As a child, my condition was controlled with the standard prescription of steroid-based ointments which can leave the skin thinned, and in many cases, permanently scarred. I was lucky, the eczema affected my arms and legs, not my face, but other sufferers are not so fortunate. Over the years I tried many alternative therapies, the most successful of which was visualisation which literally 'willed' the angry red rashes away. However, nothing proved to be a permanent cure and I became resigned to covering up with long-sleeved clothing even in the height of summer. The word eczema is from the Greek verb to boil, a good description of the chronically inflamed and intensely itchy skin. There are few conditions more demoralising than serious skin disorders that won't respond to treatment and I will admit to swallowing my first dose of evening primrose oil shrouded in a cloud of gloom. However, the effect was remarkable. Within days the itching stopped and my skin started to heal. The roughened, scaly patches that covered my arms began to fade, until after just one month they had disappeared altogether. I have taken evening primrose oil capsules on a regular basis ever since and my eczema has never returned.

Conventional medicine has yet to find a drug that effectively treats eczema and does not have damaging side-effects, yet it is one of the commonest diseases of the skin. Sufferers are driven to distraction by the overwhelming urge to scratch, which inevitably leads to severe scaling, bleeding and weeping of blisters under the skin. Not only is eczema unsightly, it is also extremely uncomfortable and frustratingly difficult to cure. The commonest form of eczema is atopic eczema, thought to be triggered by allergies, and commonest in families where there is a history of asthma and hay fever. Atopic eczema is due to a faulty immune system which leads to the body being unable to distinguish invading bacteria and viruses from harmless environmental substances such as pollen, house dust and mite droppings. Conventional medication includes steroid and antihistamine drugs, which may work for some sufferers but do have side effects and are often disappointingly ineffective. Atopic eczema is commonest amongst young children and Dr David Atherton, paediatric dermatologist at the Hospital For Sick Children, Great Ormond Street, is in no doubt of the mental as well as physical scars it leaves on the victim. He says 'in some respects it is easier and less distressing to care for a child with leukaemia than a child suffering from atopic eczema.

The disease causes unbearable physical distress for which there is often little relief.'

Children who develop atopic eczema usually do so between the ages of three and six months at the time when most are weaned. One clue that the gamma linolenic acid in evening primrose oil could be a factor in curing eczema was found when breast-fed babies who switched to solids developed the disease. Human breast milk contains GLA and breast-fed babies receive the same amount of GLA found in two to three capsules of evening primrose oil every day. Although the makers of formula feeds claim their products are as close in composition as possible to human milk, it is surprising that they do not contain any GLA at all. According to one manufacturer, adding GLA is 'unnecessary and impractical' and would reduce shelf life. However, the Japanese manage to add GLA to their formula milks by a process of micro-encapsulation. British formula milks contain linolenic acid, which should be converted by the body into GLA. However, studies show that some babies do not carry out this conversion process properly. Even purely breast-fed babies may not receive enough GLA to protect them from eczema if their mother's blood has low levels of GLA. It may therefore be sensible for lactating women to supplement their diet with evening primrose oil. While long-term trials to compare breast and formula-fed babies are currently underway, studies show that children already suffering from atopic eczema (the most common kind) have unusually low levels of unsaturated fatty acids in their bloodstream. The news that most of these children will outgrow eczema by the time they reach puberty is little consolation to those enduring the agonies of it at the time.

Having established the link between the GLA in evening primrose oil and eczema, literally hundreds of trials involving eczema sufferers have taken place. One of the most widely publicised was carried out by the department of dermatology at Bristol's Royal Infirmary and the results published in the *Lancet* report a significant improvement in patients with atopic eczema. These improvements were recorded after just three weeks of taking 4000 mg of evening primrose oil a day (2000 mg a day for children). The evening primrose oil was shown to improve itching by

36 per cent, scaling by 33 per cent and redness by 29 per cent. Similar trials at the dermatology clinic at the University of Bologna in Italy report 'substantial improvements' in the clinical symptoms of atopic eczema after four weeks of evening primrose oil therapy. Evening primrose oil is now available on prescription for the relief of atopic eczema and as children often have difficulty swallowing large capsules, it also comes in capsules with a neck that is snipped off so the oil can be squeezed on to food or into a drink. Sufferers from psoriasis also seem to benefit from taking evening primrose oil, and clinical trials report moderate improvements in 60 per cent of patients given evening primrose oil over an eight-week period.

Dry Skin
The nutritional significance of essential fatty acids such as GLA was initially highlighted in trials involving rats fed on a totally fat-free diet. The rats quickly developed skin disorders, most noticeably very dry, scaling patches of skin. We will also see similar skin disorders if we cut fat and oil from our diet completely, which is one reason why fat-free diets are so damaging. One of the many functions of the essential fatty acids in our diet is to maintain the water barrier that exists beneath the stratum corneum, or uppermost layer of skin cells. A dry, devitalised complexion is not caused by a lack of oil in the skin, but is due instead to the evaporation of water through this barrier. Therefore any holes or weakened areas in it will allow more moisture to escape and lead to excessively dry skin. GLA is an important constituent of the cellular membranes that make up this barrier, so we need to receive regular supplies to ensure that it remains stable and strong.

Pre-Menstrual Syndrome
It is thought that about 40 per cent of women worldwide suffer from some form of Pre-Menstrual Syndrome. Many sufferers first experience the symptoms of irritability and depression during their teens, while others escape until their early thirties. It affects all races and levels of society and some of the more famous sufferers include Queen Victoria, Maria Callas, Marilyn Monroe and Judy Garland. PMS can cause severe emotional upset and in 1980 two

British women separately accused of murder pleaded Pre-Menstrual Syndrome as part of their defence. As a result, both had their charges reduced to manslaughter on the grounds of diminished responsibility and were put on probation. One of the main causes of Pre-Menstrual Syndrome is the imbalance between the hormones oestrogen, progesterone and prolactin just before menstruation. An excess of prolactin in particular is linked to high stress levels and has a direct effect on breast pain, causing tenderness and swelling. These three hormones are governed by a group of prostaglandins called PGE_1, PGE_2 and PGF_2, which can cause the uterine contractions that lead to stomach cramps and water retention.

Evening primrose oil is known to affect and regulate the action of prostaglandins and has undergone extensive trials to try and pinpoint its action in relieving PMS. One such experiment, detailed in the *Pharmaceutical Journal*, took place at St Thomas's hospital in London. Sixty-eight women were involved, all of whom were classed as having severe PMS symptoms which failed to respond to conventional medication. The women were given 2000 mg of evening primrose oil a day (4 x 500 mg capsules), and at the end of the trial 61 per cent said they had total relief from PMS while 23 per cent reported partial relief. It is thought that the women suffered from low prostaglandin levels caused by poor absorption of linoleic acid or its subsequent conversion into GLA. This is quickly rectified with an evening primrose oil supplement, and by regulating the action of PGE_1, PGE_2 and PGF_2 the oil corrects the imbalances that can lead to PMS in many sufferers.

Breast Pain
Pre-menstrual breast tenderness is another complaint that responds well to treatment with evening primrose oil and patients suffering from mastalgia (severe breast pain) can now obtain the oil on prescription from their doctor. Many breast conditions are governed by the action of hormones and breast growth is stimulated during the teenage years by hormonal activity during puberty. By their early twenties, most women have reached their final bust size, although almost all will notice slight changes in breast shape and texture during their monthly cycle. It is quite

common for breasts to enlarge in the two weeks before a period, and to return to normal after the period begins. A much more visible change takes place during pregnancy, when hormones can double breast size and increase blood flow by 180 per cent. While these hormonal fluctuations are perfectly normal, some trigger other breast problems. The most common breast disorder is pre-menstrual mastalgia which affects some 5 million women in Britain between the ages of 20 and 50. Other benign (non-cancerous) breast problems include nodularity or lumpiness of the breast just before a period, and fibroadenoma, a smooth movable lump most often seen in young women. But breast pain is the commonest complaint and can affect part or all of the breast and even extend to the upper arms.

Although women with breast pain appear to have normal hormone levels, their breast tissues are unusually sensitive to hormonal actions. This increased sensitivity is linked to the pattern of essential fatty acids in the bloodstream and victims often have low levels of GLA. They may also have high levels of saturated fats that increase the effects of hormones on breast tissues and trigger pain. The first experience of mastalgia can cause the terrible fear of breast cancer. Fortunately, breast pain is rarely a symptom of cancer and is also far easier to treat. However, conventional medications are far from ideal. Painkillers and diuretics are frequently ineffective and hormone-related drugs carry their own side effects. In an attempt to find a more acceptable, natural cure for breast pain, double-blind clinical trials involving evening primrose oil were carried out at the Breast Clinic of the University of Wales. Here, a pharmaceutical quality evening primrose oil was compared to the most commonly prescribed drugs, bromocriptine and danazol. All three medications were similarly effective, but their levels of side-effects differed enormously. Only 2.2 per cent of those given the evening primrose oil experienced any side effects at all, compared to 23.6 per cent and 24.7 per cent for bromocriptine and danazol respectively. Also, the side effects for those taking the evening primrose oil formulation were much less acute, the most common being a mild stomach upset. The medical team from the Cardiff clinic reported in the *Lancet* that after reassurance about cancer, the evening primrose oil treatment should be the first line of treatment for breast pain. Their studies found that 45 per cent of patients suffering from persistent, severe breast pain benefited from the 3000 mg dose of evening primrose oil. However, as the oil works by changing the essential fatty acid composition of cell membranes it is inevitably a slow cure, and the dose must be taken every day for three to six months.

A word about breast cancer: while evening primrose oil can be effective at treating breast pain, it should not be seen as a panacea for all breast problems. Breast cancer is the biggest cause of cancer deaths in women and so it is vitally important not to confuse benign breast conditions with a potential malignancy. Breast cancer is almost non-existent among those under the age of 25, but once past this age the numbers of sufferers rise rapidly. Monthly self-examination is important for all women and any lump or change in appearance must be checked by a doctor. It is very scary discovering a breast lump, but the vast majority are benign cysts and easily removed. Fluid-filled cysts are simply drained with a fine needle and are not thought to be related in any way to breast cancer.

Multiple Sclerosis
Multiple sclerosis affects one in a thousand people in Britain and most of its sufferers are young adult women. Although the exact cause of MS is not yet known, it is believed to be an auto-immune disorder, triggered when the body's own immune system starts attacking itself. The disease affects the nervous system and begins with the destruction of the protective sheath called myelin that surrounds nerve fibres in the brain and spinal cord. The symptoms of MS include blurred vision and a tingling or numbness in the body which can lead to paralysis in later life. These symptoms vary in severity and may come and go from one week to the next, so a patient who is severely disabled one week may seem quite normal the next. While we don't know what prompts MS to strike, we do know that those with MS lack certain essential fatty acids, especially linoleic acid. This deficiency is thought to be an important factor in the degenerative nature of the disease. Studies using evening primrose oil have found its high

levels of GLA useful in preventing the immune system's white blood cells from attacking the myelin sheath and destroying the vulnerable nerve cells underneath. Some medics suggest that evening primrose oil may be more active in children suffering from MS, and that it may help if given as a protective measure to children in MS families.

MS – A Case History

Sue was 29 when multiple sclerosis struck. A previously healthy, energetic and athletic person, her first symptoms were blurred vision and dizziness. 'I woke up one morning and realised that my eyes wouldn't focus properly. When I stood up I felt very dizzy and unsteady, and I couldn't control my eyes. My neurologist recommended taking evening primrose oil from the beginning. It was also recommended by my doctor, who luckily for me is one of the more enlightened medics. I was diagnosed in May 1988, and have been taking six capsules a day ever since (each containing 430 mg evening primrose oil and 107 mg marine fish oil). I have to touch wood before I say that my symptoms have never returned and I can honestly say that I have never felt healthier. I have totally reassessed my diet and don't ever eat any saturated fat. All my oil require-ments come from the evening primrose oil capsules. I just think that you've got to start thinking about making the cellular insulation material myelin. Taking evening prim-rose oil provides the essential fatty acids for the body in the form of GLA which is like giving fat in a pre-digested form. I'm sure that if I stopped taking it my cells would be less protected and I won't take that risk. I feel much better now altogether – my cellulite has vanished and my skin has a much smoother, more youthful texture. I put it down to my revised diet and would advise any sufferer to seek advice from an informed doctor or qualified nutritionist.'

The Link with Epilepsy

Despite being under close medical scrutiny for many years, no serious side effects have been linked with taking evening primrose oil. The most common complaint is a mild stomach upset and this can usually be relieved by taking the capsules with food. Some patients also report looser bowel movements as a result of taking the oil, which is probably not a bad thing. However, there is a small but persistent claim that crops up in the popular press linking evening primrose oil with epilepsy. So is there any truth in this story that threatens to undermine its medical credentials? The link with epilepsy stems from medical trials carried out several years ago. Over three hundred people took part and three developed epilepsy during the trial. One patient was subsequently found to have been taking the placebo, so evening primrose oil could not have been the cause. The other two had been mis-diagnosed as schizophrenics, when they were in fact already suffering from epilepsy. However, because these cases came to light during the clinical trials they were mistakenly linked to the evening primrose oil. Since then, epileptics who are prescribed evening primrose oil are monitored by their doctors as a precautionary measure, but no adverse reactions have been reported to date.

The Future

Because of the effect evening primrose oil has in boosting our GLA and thus prostaglandin levels, this natural supplement has been the subject of a record amount of interest around the world. Clinical research is currently being carried out at 26 top teaching hospitals in Britain alone, focusing on the effects of essential fatty acids and their relationship with prostaglandins. Diabetes is just one disease currently under investigation using evening primrose oil therapy. Diabetics suffer from a blockage in the process that converts linoleic acid into GLA. Exactly why this occurs is not yet clear, but it seems to be linked to an imbalance of metabolic hormones and prostaglandins that regulate the release of insulin. However, initial double-blind clinical trials show that diabetic nerve damage can be repaired with 4000 mg of evening primrose oil, taken every day for a six-month period. Other clinical trials are also currently underway to assess the effect of evening primrose oil on inflammatory disorders, such as osteo- and rheumatoid arthritis and irritable bowel syndrome. Encouraging results of evening primrose oil therapy have also been seen in cases of alcohol-induced liver damage, hyperactivity in children and cystic fibrosis. Evening primrose oil may also have a stimulating effect on converting fat into energy and could be useful in treating obesity and discouraging general weight gain. Impressive results have also been reported when it is used for disorders associated with hormonal imbalances and many women suffering from menopausal problems have found evening primrose oil capsules useful. These have helped reduce the symptoms of bloating, water retention, irritability and depression. Many women already take a daily capsule or two of evening primrose oil to ward off such ailments, but do bear in mind that to have any effect on the more acute conditions previously described the dose must be increased to 2000 mg to 4000 mg every day for a *minimum of* four weeks. Whether used as an all-round tonic or specific treatment for more serious disorders, the on-going medical interest in evening primrose oil will no doubt ensure that this humble herb plays an increasingly important role in health protection.

Linseed Oil (Linum usitatissumum)

The History

Linseed oil takes its name from the Latin for most useful and comes from the flax plant. Flax is an annual crop with rich blue flowers and tiny brownish yellow seeds. There are several different varieties, each with different uses. The long-stemmed variety is grown for its lengthy fibres that are woven into linen. While the short-stemmed varieties tend to concentrate their goodness in the seeds and are used for oil extraction. Flax needs a rich, wet soil with plenty of hand labour and is an important crop in Northern Ireland where it is used to make Irish linen. The oil-laden seeds are warm-pressed to extract the oil, and several organically grown varieties are now available.

The use of linseed oil can be traced back to Hippocrates who recorded that it was a useful treatment for stomach and skin disorders. More recent advocates of linseed oil include Mahatma Gandhi who wrote: 'Whenever flax seed becomes a regular food item among the people there will be better health.' Linseed is valued by herbalists for its mucilage properties, meaning it contains a slimy material that is not absorbed but passes straight through the body.

Linseeds are a very effective and gentle bulking agent and can be used as a laxative when swallowed whole with plenty of water. The mucins and water-binding substances in the linseeds work by increasing the volume of the stool. This then presses against the intestinal walls and triggers the action of peristalsis (intestinal movement). In addition, the mucins form a protective and gliding film which covers the sensitive mucous membranes. This can then help heal any intestinal wall irritation. Crushed linseeds are also used in poultices and have the ability to draw out excess fluid from body tissues. Linseed poultices are used to treat the swollen fetlocks of racehorses and help heal altfetic injuries. Some aromatherapists also use them in conjunction with massage to tighten slack skin tissues and combat cellulite. Today, linseed oil is used mainly by paint manufacturers and sold as a conditioning oil for cricket bats. However, following the discovery of its essential fatty acid content, linseed oil is making a timely nutritional come-back.

The Science

Of all the seeds used for oil extraction, linseeds give up their oil with the least struggle and the oil accounts for over half their weight. Although a relative newcomer on the market, linseed oil contains mainly Omega-3, and some Omega-6 and Omega-9 fatty acids. It is a rich natural source of the Omega-3 essential fatty acid called alpha linolenic acid (ALA) which can, to a small extent, be converted by the body into EPA and DHA. These are the Omega-3 polyunsaturates found in fish oils. Linseed oil has therefore been recommended for vegetarians who prefer not to take fish oils. However, research has shown that this conversion process is limited. In addition to its high levels of essential fatty acids, linseed oil also contains beta carotene (the most potent precursor of vitamin A) and vitamin E.

Health Benefits

Some of the most extraordinary work with cancer patients has focused on using linseed oil. Dr Johanna Budwig is a biochemist and nutritionist in West Germany and has long believed in the use of unrefined oils to promote good health. Her unusual dietary regime involves taking 120 ml (8 tablespoonfuls) of linseed oil in 100 g (4 oz) of cottage cheese every day. Dr Budwig's theory is that the sulphur-rich proteins in the cottage cheese help ensure the essential fatty acids in the oil are utilised properly in the body. She says: 'It is obvious that if we feed the body the highly unsaturated essential fatty acids it requires, along with the high quality protein which makes the fat easily soluble, and if we also stay away from chemical preservatives, then many, many people will become healthy very fast. I have proved this premise many times.' Dr Budwig claims to have over 1000 documented cases of successful cancer treatment using linseed oil, and her controversial work has been repeatedly nominated for the Nobel Prize in medicine. However, with such a difficult and emotive disease as cancer, it is clear that more research needs to be carried out to assess the true value of linseed oil.

One of the drawbacks to linseed oil is that it needs to be used fresh as it spoils much faster than other oils. Even when kept cool and tightly sealed linseed oil looses its nutrients after four months. Light, air and high tempera-tures destroy its Omega-3 alpha linolenic acid very rapidly, and linseed oil should be kept in the fridge and used within six weeks of opening. However, linseed oil is also available in capsule form which protects the oil from spoilage. When buying the liquid oil, choose one that has been packed in a light-proof container. Because of its short shelf life, the best varieties carry both the date the oil was extracted and a best-before date. Linseed oil has a peculiar, organic taste and is best used in salad dressings or added to milkshakes. It can also be blended with other oils such as olive oil to boost their nutritional value.

Olive Oil (Olea europea)

The History

Olive oil is the king of oils and has legendary health and beauty properties. Since the early days of mankind, the olive tree has been a powerful symbol of strength, peace and fertility. The Ancient Egyptians were amongst the first to use olive oil, regarding it as a gift from their great goddess Isis. Large casks of olive oil were entombed alongside the pharoahs and garlands of olive branches were found crowning the head of Tutankhamun.

The Ancient Greeks also valued olive oil, believing it to be a gift from Athena, whilst the Hebrews have valued the olive tree since Adam. The Bible contains some of the earliest references to the olive – from the Book of Exodus where Moses is told how to make an anointing oil from spiced olives to Noah's dove returning to the ark clutching an olive branch in its beak. Early civilisations used olive oil as a form of currency and it provided fuel for their lamps as well as being a food and medicine. Homer referred to olive oil as liquid gold and the fathers of medicine, Hippocrates and Galen, prescribed it for sunburn. Pedacius Dioscorides, who wrote one of the first manuscripts on herbal medicine during the 1st century AD, also used olive oil to treat stomach disorders.

The Science

Spain is the world's leading olive grower and has some 200 million trees producing between 450,000 and 750,000 metric tons of olive oil every year. The olives grown for pressing are soft and squashy, unlike the firmer varieties grown for the table. There are about 60 different oil-bearing varieties, all of which are green at first and turn black as they ripen. Although it takes up to 10 years before an olive tree bears its first fruit, it is long-lived and can flourish for 600 years or more. There are four principal olive oil regions in Spain and each produces an oil which differs in flavour and appearance from the rest. Because their flavours are so diverse, the oils from these areas are awarded Labels of Origin which state where the olives were grown and whether the oil is the result of an early harvest (slightly bitter) or a late harvest (paler and sweeter). Olive oil varies in taste and colour from year to year depending on the variety of olives used and the time of harvesting. Like a fine wine, the taste also depends largely on the climate and growing conditions, but unlike a vintage claret, olive oil doesn't improve with age.

Olive oil labels can be read in the same way as wine labels to reveal the quality and taste of their contents. The best Spanish oils come from Borjas Blancas, Siurana, Baena and Sierra de Segura. All four areas produce the best quality extra virgin olive oils, classified as having less than 1 per cent acidity.

Compared to other nut and seed oils, olive oil is one of the simplest to process. It was originally extracted by crushing olives in hessian bags suspended in barrels of water. When the oil floated to the top of the barrels it was skimmed off and bottled. Nowadays most olive oil is extracted by cold-pressing, and it is still the easiest type of oil to find in its raw, unrefined state. Virgin olive oil is classified as the unrefined juice of the fruit with an acidity level of less than 2 per cent. Extra virgin olive oil has an acidity level of less than 1 per cent and is the best – and most expensive – type you can buy. Bottles labelled 'pure' olive oil are not as unadulterated as their name implies and contain a blend of both refined and virgin olive oils. Supermarket own-labels and well-known brands may be extracted using a combination of heat and solvents, and are mixed to a standard recipe so they taste the same every time. The most pungent, full-flavoured olive oils are dark green in colour and their powerful aromas are best suited for sparing use in dressings and sauces. Olive oil is one of the longest lasting oils as it forms fewer of the degenerating peroxides that cause rancidity when exposed to heat or daylight. Unlike some cooking oils, olive oil produces fewer of the dangerous peroxides and aldehydes that have toxic effects in the body. So for those who still insist on the occasional fry-up, olive oil is the best type of oil to choose as its chemical structure remains the most stable at high temperatures. In cooking terms at least, olive oil has the fewest number of negative factors and the greatest number of health-giving properties.

Health Benefits

The link between olive oil and heart disease was first discovered by scientists at the University of Minnesota who undertook an extensive study into the worldwide numbers of deaths from heart disease. They discovered that the death rates were lowest amongst those whose main source of dietary fat is olive oil. One of the lowest incidences of heart disease is in Crete where the oil flows like wine and its native population receive up to half their calorific intake from olive oil alone. Not only do they cook exclusively with the stuff, the Cretans also knock back a glass or two as a preprandial aperitif. The Italians are also great consumers of olive oil and their incidence of heart disease is correspondingly low. The effects of olive oil on the system are certainly impressive and just two-thirds of a tablespoonful taken every day has been shown to lower blood pressure. Some doctors in Milan actually prescribe a daily dose of 60–75 ml (4–5 tablespoonfuls) of olive oil to patients suffering from heart disease and thrombosis.

The reason olive oil has such a potent effect within the body lies within its chemical composition. Olive oil is dominated by monounsaturated fatty acids which alter the overall cholesterol balance in the bloodstream in a more beneficial way than polyunsaturated vegetable oils. This is because olive oil lowers our total cholesterol levels while preserving the beneficial HDL type of cholesterol. This action preserves the important protective ratios of HDLs to LDLs, in contrast to that of the polyunsaturated fats which knock out both good and bad forms of cholesterol. Olive oil is now widely regarded as being as effective at combating high cholesterol levels as a low-fat diet, although too much saturated fat from meat and dairy products will block its health-giving action.

In addition to monounsaturated fatty acids, olive oil also contains over a thousand active chemical compounds, many of which are currently under investigation. One chemical, called cycloarthanol, seems to play a particularly important part in preventing the absorption of excess cholesterol in the body. Olive oil has also been found to have a similar ratio of essential fatty acids as human breast milk and is a good oil to use when preparing foods for small children. It is also a source of vitamin E which protects the body against harmful free-radical cell damage. Other benefits from olive oil include anti-coagulating agents that thin the blood and reduce the risk of blood clotting. It also strengthens the delicate membranes surrounding our cells and makes them less susceptible to free-radical damage.

Olive oil has traditionally been used for stomach disorders and we now know that it stimulates bile production and will encourage the gall bladder to contract, reducing the risk of gall stones. It also promotes pancreatic secretions and may even protect against stomach ulcers.

Oil of Javanicus

Future Potential

The most recent oil supplement does not come from nuts or seeds, but was created in the laboratory by an age-old fermentation process. Called Oil of Javanicus, it is one of the richest sources of gamma linolenic acid and contains 16 per cent pure GLA. This figure beats evening primrose oil which contains about 9 per cent pure GLA.

The micro-organisms used to create Oil of Javanicus were first discovered by a German scientist, C. Wehmer, as long ago as 1900. Wehmer discovered the organisms in a starter culture used by Indonesians to create tempeh, a fermented food from soya beans which is a staple of the Indonesian diet. Over 70,000 tons of soya beans are turned into tempeh each year. The micro-organisms used in the fermentation process are called *Mucor javanicus* and they give the oil its unusual name. It wasn't until 1965, however, that *Mucor javanicus* was found to be capable of creating GLA. Following the medical discoveries of the health benefits from the GLA in evening primrose oil, a biotechnology programme was set up at Hull University to find a fermentation process which could produce a suitable carrying medium, such as an oil. The programme started in 1976 and was run by Professor Colin Ratledge, who specialises in finding sources of GLA produced by fungi. From laboratory culture to full-scale production took eight years, including the time to carry out the neccessary safety trials to ensure that the oil really was as good as the scientists had hoped. In the same way that micro-organisms used for beer and wine-making convert sugar into alcohol, *Mucor javanicus* transforms glucose into an oil rich in GLA.

Oil of Javanicus falls into the category of a single cell oil, a jargon phrase adopted by scientists to cover any oil grown from micro-organisms. Single cell oils appear to have many distinct advantages over plant oils such as evening primrose oil and borage oil. Because they are grown in the laboratory, they can be produced to a consistently high specification, without the worry of undesirable treatments such as herbicides and pesticides. Professor Ratledge (who is passionate on the subject) refers to single cell oils as being clean and absolutely pure. They are certainly easier to produce as they are not subject to the vagaries of the weather, soil conditions or crop diseases. All of these factors can adversely affect the quality and quantity of the fatty acids in seed oils. This element of ultimate quality control could make single cell oils especially valuable to the pharmaceutical industry, where some prescription-only medications rely on precise quantities of GLA. At the moment, however, only evening primrose oil holds a medical licence not GLA, despite this fatty acid being the active ingredient. If GLA were to become a prescribable medicine in its own right, the flood gates would open and the pharmaceutical giants would almost certainly turn to biotechnology as their principal source.

As single cell oils are easier to produce they should also cost the consumer less and when Oil of Javanicus was on the market it cost about half the price of evening primrose oil. So why is it that in view of its many benefits Oil of Javanicus is not a household name? Despite a lengthy PR campaign, the oil singularly failed to capture the imagination of the buying public and as a result has been withdrawn from sale. However, its development was far from a wasted exercise and the biotechnology behind it still exists for future use. What the scientific and medical world has to decide is whether single cell oils as a concept are commercially viable or simply academic curiosities. Perhaps when the full benefits of GLA have been uncovered in the years to come, we will return to this futuristic oil for the simplest answer to many complex health problems.

3

The Vital Oils Beauty Diet

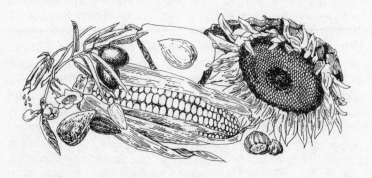

The health benefits of oils are well known but they are also important for our looks too. Unrefined vegetable oils are a good source of essential fatty acids and vitamins – the nutrients needed to improve the condition of our skin, hair and nails. When taken internally, either in the diet or in the form of capsule supplements, these oils supply our skin cells with the essential fatty acids and vitamins needed to maintain healthy cell membranes. Essential fatty acids are an important component of the delicate membranes that surround every cell in the body. By increasing their strength, our skin cells become better able to ward off attacks from the destructive enzymes and other elements that provoke skin ageing. Many oils also contain useful levels of vitamins A and E, often referred to as the skincare nutrients for their regenerative and protective powers. Vitamin A is needed to maintain healthy skin tissues and skin tone, while vitamin E is an antioxidant and protects against the free-radical cell damage that is widely believed to be the major force in ageing. By increasing the amount of oil in our diet, we can not only improve our appearance but can also help delay the fine lines and wrinkles.

In addition, there are many other important benefits to be gained from following the *Vital Oils Beauty Diet*. It has been devised to boost energy levels, improve overall good health and will also help you lose weight. Oils are relatively high-calorie, energy-giving foods, so how can they help us slim? The answer is to revise the type of oils we eat, and to cut out the over-refined and saturated kind that overload the body and clog up the system. Oil supplements are also a very useful way of increasing your daily oil intake and are remarkably low in calories. The average beauty oil capsule, such as avocado oil, contains just 3 Kcal (12.5 kJ) each.

The good news is that the *Vital Oils Beauty Diet* does not insist you count calories, but it does follow the proven, commonsense guidelines of reducing saturated fats, sugars and salt while increasing fibre. In fact, this oil-enriched food plan combines sensible eating with tasty and filling foods. Oils can be quickly converted into energy by the body so these recipes will keep your vitality levels high. This is also an eating plan which will never leave you feeling hungry, as increasing the amount of fibre from raw fruits and vegetables, wholegrain breads, pasta, rice, beans and nuts will produce a steadier and more prolonged supply of blood sugar energy. This simple regime will also improve a sluggish elimination system and encourage the body to get rid of toxins faster.

The first step of the *Vital Oils Beauty Diet* is to go through your shopping list and strike off the saturated fats. These block the actions of the cold-pressed vegetable and nut oils used in the recipes and have no place in a health and beauty weight-loss regime. Definite results will be seen by avoiding cream, lard and suet and by reducing red meats and dairy products such as full-fat milk and cheese. As we have already seen, highly refined oils may not be as beneficial to our health as we are led to believe, so all the oils specified in the recipes are raw and unrefined. Butter and hard margarines are high in saturated fats so should be avoided, and although high polyunsaturated spreads are made with polyunsaturates, their structure is usually changed by a process called hydrogenation. In this process hydrogen is bonded into the oil molecules to change their structure from a liquid into a solid fat. Hydrogenation destroys the health benefits of the oils, so it is worth seeking out unhydrogenated spreads from health food shops. Although the *Vital Oils Beauty Diet* is not strictly vegetarian, the emphasis is on fresh, natural produce with plenty of fruit and vegetables, wholegrains, beans, nuts and seeds, with some chicken. A regular intake of fish oils is also highly beneficial and so there are also recipes using oily fish such as mackerel, trout, tuna and anchovy. None of the foods are naturally high in calories either, just avoid the saturated fats or sugars that traditionally accompany them.

Most diets don't work because they are too hard to follow, so this is not a strict eating plan. The *Vital Oils Beauty Diet* is infinitely variable and each day can be adapted or swapped to suit your own lifestyle, working or shopping arrangements. The tried-and-tested recipes have been created to fit in with busy lives and are easily scaled down for single portions or adjusted to feed a large, hungry family. Often, the starter for dinner is served the following day for lunch and this saves time and effort, especially for those going out to work. A large, mixed salad can be swapped for any meal you don't fancy or haven't the time to make. You will also find some of my personal favourites which will add variety to the diet plan. You can be flexible – but do use 15 ml (1 table-spoonful) of unrefined, uncooked oil in one meal per day. As we have seen, all oils aren't created equal though, so only use the oils mentioned to see maximum health and beauty benefits. All are easily available and include virgin olive oil, safflower, sesame seed and sunflower oil. The more unusual varieties such as walnut and hazelnut oil can be found in health food shops or delicatessens.

After following the *Vital Oils Beauty Diet* for just four weeks you can expect to see the following improvements:

– Improved skin, hair and nail condition.
– Higher energy levels and increased vitality
– Less PMS and menopausal symptoms
– Strengthened immunity to invading viruses and bacteria
– Better digestion and elimination
– Reduced allergy symptoms
– Improvements in inflammatory disorders such as arthritis.

General Guidelines

- Cut down on stimulants such as tea, coffee and cola drinks. Substitute with fresh fruit and vegetable juices (diluted with filtered water or low-salt mineral water). Fruit and herb teas plus plenty of pure water (at least six large glasses daily) will also speed the elimination of toxins.
- Use lower fat skimmed or semi-skimmed milk.
- Beware of high-fat dressings and mayonnaise and only use low-fat versions in moderation.
- If you get hunger pangs between meals, snack on fibrous fruits such as apples, pears, oranges and grapes. These will cleanse and refresh the palate as well as stave off hunger attacks.

A word on weight-reduction: A slow, steady weight-loss is the best way to lose extra pounds and keep them off permanently. When you have completed the first two weeks of the eating plan, repeat, substituting your own favourite ingredients or dishes within the guidelines. When the four weeks are over, don't revert to rich or over-refined foods or you will undo all the good work. You will continue to notice health and beauty benefits if you simply allow the basics of the *Vital Oils Beauty Diet* diet to become part of your life. Remember, the food we eat not only gives us the energy to work, exercise and sleep well, but it also determines the quality of our skin, hair, blood, bones, muscles – in fact every possible part of us. It also helps to ensure that having gained our good looks, we keep them for far longer too, so it has to be worth just a little extra thought and effort.

A Guide To Cooking Oils

Pure, unrefined cooking oils are more expensive than the processed blends, but they taste far better and contain many important nutrients such as vitamin E and lecithin. None of the recipes in the *Vital Oils Beauty Diet* involves using large quantities of oil, eg for deep-frying, and it is more a question of using small amounts of the best quality oils to achieve better health. All unrefined oils have their own natural flavours and you can play around with the different varieties to suit your tastebuds and your pocket.

The cooking guide below includes grapeseed, rapeseed, groundnut and soybean oils, although I have yet to find them in unrefined versions. However, they are also the cheapest cooking oils and the information given below is intended to help you decide which best suit your taste and budget. As a general rule, all oils should be stored away from strong light, so only buy from shops that have a rapid turnover and have not left them on the shelves for months on end.

Corn Oil (zea mays)

Corn or maize oil is high in polyunsaturates and is one of the cheapest, most commonly used oils for cooking. Corn oil comes from the corn-on-the-cob plant and is extracted from the sweetcorn kernels. Most corn oil comes from America and southern France where it is usually heavily refined for blended cooking oils. However it is possible to find pure, unrefined versions in health food shops. Unrefined corn oil contains useful levels of the natural antioxidant vitamin E (66 mg per 100 g). Being a polyunsaturated oil, it is a good source of the Omega-6 essential fatty acids. Corn oil deteriorates when heated to high temperatures, so is best kept for recipes that use it cold or warm, such as sauces. Some cooks consider corn oil to be too heavy to use in salad dressings. Also, as a polyunsaturated oil, it needs protecting from heat, light and exposure to the air. It is best bought in small quantities so you use it up faster and should be stored in the fridge. Inexpensive dressings can be made using corn oil as a base with small quantities of the more expensive nut oils added for flavour.

Grapeseed Oil (vitis vinifera)

Grapeseed oil comes from grape pips and, not surprisingly, most of the oil we import comes from the wine-growing regions of France. Although the grapevine has been around for thousands of years, commercial oil extraction is a fairly new process. Grapeseed oil has one of the highest polyunsaturated fatty acid contents, second only to safflower. Unrefined grapeseed oil is considered unpalatable and is not available on the general market. Refined grapeseed oil is light and tasteless and useful as a neutral base for salad dressings to which more nutritious oils are added. Because it has a fine texture and no smell, grapeseed oil is also useful as a massage oil. It has a high smoke point which means that it can be heated to higher temperatures before giving off a bluish coloured smoke. An oil's smoke point is influenced by the presence of free fatty acids and crude oils that contain larger quantities of free fatty acids have a lower smoke point. When an oil starts to smoke it is a sign that it has started to break down and should be discarded.

Groundnut Oil (arachis hypogaea)

Groundnut oil is another name for peanut oil and comes from peanut kernels. The peanut plant belongs to the same legume family as the soya bean. It is a hardy annual that thrives on a light soil and subtropical climate, is fast growing and will produce its first crop of peanuts just four months after planting. The peanut plant is mainly cultivated in undeveloped countries as it can be harvested by hand. It is an important crop in Nigeria and other parts of West Africa and in China, South America and India. Technically the kernels are not nuts at all but seed pods that develop underground. Peanuts in their raw state are highly nutritious and consist of about 45 per cent oil, 30 per cent protein and valuable quantities of iron, vitamin B (niacin) and vitamin E. Peanuts are best eaten straight from their shells and much of their nutritional benefit may be lost when processed as 'dry-roasted' snacks.

Groundnut oil is usually highly refined and also loses many of its healthy attributes in processing. In its raw state it is a useful source of vitamin E (21 mg per 100 ml). It is a monounsaturated oil which also has a high level of polyunsaturated fatty acids. As with rapeseed and soybean oils, groundnut oil has a high smoke point so is often recommended for shallow frying.

Hazelnut Oil (corylus avellana)

Although this is the newest vegetable oil to appear in the supermarket, hazelnut oil is first thought to have been extracted during the Bronze Age. Hazelnuts, also known as cobnuts or filberts, originate from a tall shrub that grows wild throughout Europe. These nuts are a nutritious food, being the lowest of the nuts in fat and containing useful levels of vitamin E. Hazelnut oil is most commonly warm-pressed from the small nut kernels. After pressing, the hazelnut oil is left to settle in vats where it takes about a week for the sediment to separate and sink to the bottom. On average, 2.5 kilos (5½ lb) of hazelnuts will yield about 1 litre (1¾ pints) of oil. Hazelnut oil is monounsaturated so can be gently heated without damaging its chemical structure. The best quality hazelnut oils are hand-produced and come from France, where gourmet cooks praise it for its sweet, smooth flavour. However, it is one of the more expensive oils, so is best used in small amounts to flavour salad dressings and sauces. Hazelnut oil is also wonderful for baking and a few drops added to nutty cake and biscuit mixtures give a deliciously subtle taste. Store in a cool, dark place. Hazelnut oil will keep for up to a year while sealed. Once open, store in the fridge.

Olive Oil (olea europaea)

Olive oil is highly versatile and was the first type of oil used for cooking. The Ancient Egyptians prized it highly not only for culinary purposes, but also for use in their sacrificial ceremonies. Most olive oil now comes from Spain, Italy, Greece and southern France, where the plentiful Mediterranean sunshine, moderate rain and enriched soil suits the cultivated olive tree. Each tree produces 10–20 kilos (22–44 lb) of olives a year and the oil is usually pressed in local olive mills located near the groves. Olive oil is very easy to find in its raw, unrefined state and most supermarkets stock cold-pressed varieties. Look for the words virgin or extra virgin on the label, which refer to the oil's quality and are also a guarantee that the oil has not been refined. Olive oil is a monounsaturated oil with low levels of vitamin E (5 mg per 100 ml). It is the most versatile of all cooking oils and can be used at high temperatures with less risk of spoilage. Olive oil also keeps well, provided it is protected from the light and heat. One of the most economical ways to buy it is in metal drums, but be sure you can tightly reseal the container or decant into smaller bottles, as exposure to the air will encourage rancidity.

Rapeseed Oil (brassica napus)

Rapeseed oil is another vegetable oil used in commercial food preparation and the refined oil has recently appeared on supermarket shelves. The rape plant belongs to the cabbage family and grows to 1.5–1.8 metres (5–6 feet) high with vivid yellow flowers. Fields of these intense yellow flowers appear from May onwards and have become a familiar landmark in the British countryside. Rape is a favourite crop with British farmers because it forms humus which feeds the tiny soil animals that keep the ground healthy. It also gives the soil a much needed break from growing wheat. Another reason for its popularity is the large EC farming subsidies for growing high-protein seed oil crops.

Rape is certainly a versatile crop. The seeds contain 35–40 per cent pure oil, and the young leaves can be served as a vegetable. The oil is used for commercial and domestic cooking, and also as an industrial lubricant. The French have also found a way of turning rapeseed oil into a less polluting form of diesel fuel, but the process is currently too expensive to be commercially viable. Both the plant and seedcake left over from the oil-refining process are popular cattle feeds. Rape grows well all over Britain, but especially in Scotland as it favours a heavy soil and long summer days. Because of its unfortunate name, some prefer to call rape cole and have renamed rapeseed coleseed. The Canadians have gone one step further and renamed their rapeseed oil Canola oil and this name has been registered as a national brand trademark.

Rapeseed oil has the highest percentage of unsaturated fats of any vegetable oil. It contains over 90 per cent mono- and polyunsaturates and is a light oil with no flavour. However, despite its valuable fatty acid content and the fact that it is a cheap, British product, rapeseed oil has a number of culinary drawbacks. Firstly, it is only available in a highly refined state and as such is devoid of many important nutrients. Also, although it has a high smoke point rapeseed oil is less stable than many other oils at high temperatures and will produce more toxic effluents when cooked. Rapeseed oil does have a high smoke point, however. On balance, rapeseed oil is a good basic oil that is best used cold or warm. It can be flavoured with a few drops of the more expensive nut oils to make it more interesting in recipes. Rapeseed oil must be protected from light and heat to delay rancidity and is best stored in the fridge.

Safflower Oil (carthamus tinctorius)

The safflower belongs to the thistle family and originates from India. It grows up to 1¼ metres (4 feet) high and was originally cultivated for its reddish flowers which were used to dye cloth vibrant shades of orange and pink. The bitter safflower fruit was also used as a red vegetable dye and this was favoured by the Ancient Egyptians for dyeing the cotton swaddling used for mummification. The safflower is now grown worldwide for the oil that can be extracted from its crop of tiny seeds.

Because safflower is cheap and easy to grow, it has become increasingly popular as a low-saturate cooking oil. High in polyunsaturates, unrefined safflower oil is rich in the Omega-6 group of essential fatty acids. Unrefined safflower oil is also a good source of vitamin E (49 mg per 100 ml). The unrefined oil has a rich, golden colour and it is possible to find organically grown versions. Safflower oil has an attractive, nutty taste and is excellent in salad dressings. However, it is one of the least stable oils at high temperatures, so should not be used for frying. It is also the most difficult vegetable oil to keep fresh, and should always be stored in the fridge.

Sesame Oil (sesamum indicum)

Sesame oil was used in cooking as far back as Roman times. The sesame plant grows to about 2 metres (over 6 feet) high and resembles garden mint. Its sweet-smelling funnel-shaped flowers are a vivid shade of pink and highly prized by the perfume industry. The sesame plant bears small nuts about an inch long, each covered with hooks to snag the coats of grazing animals and ensure seed dispersal. The seeds are contained within the nut which is divided into four tiny compartments crammed with seeds. Sesame oil is used in the manufacture of some margarines and in its unrefined state is one of the most versatile cooking oils. Being a monounsaturated oil, it can be heated to higher temperatures than polyunsaturated oils without forming toxic elements. Sesame oil may also be heated and sold as toasted sesame oil. This has a wonderfully pungent flavour and just a few drops add zest to salad dressings and marinades. However, most of its nutrients are lost in the toasting process. Both types of sesame oil should be stored in a cool, dry place. Sesame seeds themselves are a tasty source of iron, calcium and protein and can be crushed to make the oily paste tahini. They are also used to make the Greek sweetmeat called halva, a nutritious form of fudge.

Soybean Oil (glycine max)

Soybean oil is a relative newcomer to the cooking oil market, although it has a long and illustrious culinary history. Soybean oil comes from the soya plant which belongs to the pea or legume family. It can be traced back 5000 years to its first recorded cultivation in mainland China. Now there are over 1000 different varieties of the soya plant, ranging from small bushy shrubs to tall, leafy plants. Soya beans are principally grown in China, Japan, America and Brazil. The plants are unusual in that they must spend a certain length of time in complete darkness in order to flower and germinate. For this reason, soya beans are impossible to grow in places of northern latitudes (such as Britain) that have relatively short summer nights.

The oil is extracted from smooth egg-shaped beans which are usually yellow but may be black or green in colour. Their oil content is low (13–20 per cent) and for reasons of economy must be extracted with solvents. Although soybean oil is one of our cheapest cooking oils, it is almost impossible to find it in an unrefined state. When unrefined, soybean oil is our second-best source of vitamin E (87 mg per 100 ml) after wheatgerm oil and contains more lecithin than any other vegetable oil. Soybean oil has a high level of polyunsaturates and so produces toxic elements when heated at high temperatures. As with rapeseed oil, soybean oil has a high smoke point but should not be used for frying. The oil can be used and stored in the same way as rapeseed oil.

The reasons why soybean oil is so nutritious stem from the intriguing soya bean itself which deserves a special mention. Soya beans must be the world's most nutritious and versatile source of food, and in China they are nicknamed meat without bones. Not only do they have a commercially viable oil content, but they are also one of the very best sources of vegetable protein. Soya beans are widely used in vegetarian and macrobiotic cookery and can be processed to create several different types of food. Soya beans can be coagulated with nigami paste (a calcium suspension) to make tofu. This is a solid curd-type cheese with a multitude of sweet and savoury uses. Tofu is a wonderful high-protein, low-cost and low-calorie food which is easily available in health food stores. Soya beans can also be turned into tempeh, produced by boiling and dehulling soya beans and injecting them with the micro-organism *Mucor javanicus*. After a day or so, the mixture turns into a cake of fermented soya beans held together with the mycelium grown from the micro-organisms. Tempeh has a firm, mushroom-like consistency and is a staple food of the Indonesians. It is rich in protein, fibre, vitamins, Omega-3 and Omega-6 essential fatty acids. Tempeh is one of our few dietary sources of GLA and is increasingly available in health food stores. It can be eaten raw or cooked like meat, and is delicious marinated in walnut oil and baked in the oven.

Soya beans can also be crushed and blended with water to make soya milk. A light, nutty liquid, this is good for vegans or those with a lactose-intolerance and can be used in place of cow's milk. Soya milk contains more protein and iron than cow's milk and has lower levels of saturated fat, salt and fewer calories. However, it contains far less calcium than cow's milk and has a relatively high aluminium content. Another important use for soya beans is soy sauce. This famous Chinese condiment dates back to before the birth of Christ and is made with the liquid from fermented soya beans. There are two types of soy sauce, Shoyu which is made from soybeans and wheat flour, and Tamari which comes from soybeans only. Both have a high salt content (approx 440 mg of sodium per teaspoonful) and must be used sparingly. Tamari soy sauce has a stronger flavour and is the more expensive of the two. Soya beans can also be fermented to produce miso, a natural flavouring which is good to use instead of stock cubes as most contain hydrogenated vegetable oils.

Sunflower Oil (helianthus anuus)

The sunflower first appeared in Mexico and Peru and its botanical name comes from the Greek word *helios*, meaning the sun. Sunflowers can grow to 3.6 metres (12 feet) high and have a large circular seed head surrounded by soft yellow petals that resemble the sun's rays. They were an important plant to the Aztecs who worshipped the sun, and they forged replicas of the flower in gold to line their temple walls. Sunflowers are extremely fast growing and will thrive on poor soil provided they get several hours of full sunshine. The roots of the sunflower plant are highly efficient at sucking water out of the soil and sunflowers are often planted in areas that require drainage – large areas of the Netherlands are planted with sunflowers. It is a versatile plant and every part of it can be used. The petals can be steeped in water to make a yellow hair dye, the woody stalks are used in paper making and the oil is extracted from the seeds. The principal sunflower-oil-producing countries are Russia, Rumania, Hungary, Argentina, France, Australia and South Africa.

Sunflower oil is light and slightly sweet. It is extracted from the sunflower seeds as soon as they have fully ripened and turned black. The seeds contain about 40 per cent oil and are also delicious eaten raw. They make a nourishing snack and are a good source of calcium, protein, vitamins B1, B6 and potassium. Sunflower seeds can be sprouted on damp blotting paper and make a nutritious filler for salads. Sunflower oil is very high in polyunsaturates and when unrefined contains useful amounts of Omega-6 EFAs. The natural oil also contains relatively high levels of vitamin E (27 mg per 100 ml). Sunflower oil is used extensively in blended cooking oils, unfortunately most of these are highly processed and low in nutrients. However, the unrefined versions are inexpensive and easily available from health food stores. Sunflower oil is best used cold or at low temperatures as it breaks down and produces toxic elements when heated to high temperatures. It should be stored in the fridge.

Butter or Sunflower Spread?

About half of the entire sunflower oil crop is bought by the food industry for making margarine and low-fat spreads. These were originally developed during the Second World War as a cheap alternative to butter and have remained an important part of our diet. However, there is so much confusion and controversy surrounding what we should be spreading on our bread that it is well worth taking a quick look at the issues involved.

The butter v. margarine and low-fat spread debate looks set to rage well into the 21st century. Butter is relatively high in saturated fat but is favoured by some for being a pure, natural product. Margarines and low-fat spreads are highly processed products made with complicated chemical wizardry. Since the discovery that polyunsaturates are better for us than saturates, many soft margarines based on sunflower oil have appeared on the market. If a margarine spread makes any claim about polyunsaturates on the label it must satisfy strict food labelling laws. At least 45 per cent of its fat content must be polyunsaturated and not more than 25 per cent can be saturated. While these sunflower spreads are a useful source of polyunsaturates, they have about the same number of calories as butter and should not be confused with low-fat spreads. These are far lower in calories and consist of half fat and half water, but much of their fat is the saturated variety. So although low-fat spreads contain fewer calories, their fat content is less desirable for overall health. So which is better for us? This is a question which vexes nutritionists and one to which there is no easy answer. Both soft margarines and low-fat spreads invariably contain hydrogenated vegetable oil which has had its structure altered so that it behaves like a saturated fat in the body. Therefore neither is particularly desirable. If you really want a spread-from-the-fridge product, my answer is to track down an unhydrogenated spread from a health food shop or make your own by blending softened butter with unrefined sunflower oil.

Walnut Oil (juglans regia)

Walnut oil is a relative newcomer to Britain, but features strongly in even quite basic French cooking. Traditionally, French chefs use a few drops of walnut oil to fry eggs. Although America is the largest producer of walnuts, followed by China and Turkey, most of our walnut oil comes from France with the main areas of production around Perigord, the Dordogne and the Loire. Oil extraction is a time-consuming process as the shells have to be removed by hand, using a small mallet on a stone base, taking care not to break the kernel. The kernels are then ground using a millstone and warm-pressed to release the oil. After pressing, the topaz-coloured oil is filtered through cotton cloth or paper before bottling. It takes about 2 kilos (4½ lb) of walnuts to produce 1 litre (1¾ pints) of walnut oil. The oil is easy to find in its natural, unrefined state and is stocked in an increasing number of supermarkets. You will sometimes find it with its French label, Huile de Noix or Huile de Noix Extra (a slightly stronger flavour). Walnut oil is polyunsaturated and also contains low levels of GLA, and is best used cold in dressings and sauces. Although it is more expensive than other oils, a few drops go a long way and it makes a tasty addition to many recipes. As an example, try adding a few drops to walnut cookies to enhance the flavour. Unopened walnut oil keeps for up to a year if stored away from the light, but once open it is best kept in the fridge.

The Diet Plan

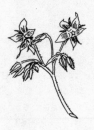

Day 1 – Monday

Breakfast
Super Breakfast Shake (see recipe)

Light Meal
Open sandwich – lettuce, mayonnaise, smoked fish, cucumber, lemon wedge

Main Meal
Jacket potato – ratatouille topping and a large mixed salad
Walnut and mustard dressing (see recipe)

Day 2 – Tuesday

Breakfast
Unsweetened fruit juice (diluted)
Scrambled egg on granary toast

Light Meal
Vegetable crudités – fromage frais flavoured with a little tomato purée or mustard, with wholemeal pitta bread
Apple, pear or banana

Main Meal
Vegetables with Dhal Sauce and Wholegrain Rice (see recipe)
Fresh fruit

Day 3 – Wednesday

Breakfast
Grilled tomatoes on toast

Light Meal
Lunchtime Salad Platter (see recipe)

Main Meal
Anchovy and Lentil Pâté (see recipe)
Omelette – mushroom, tomato or sweetcorn filling with large green salad and crusty bread
Fresh fruit

Day 4 – Thursday

Breakfast
Banana, grapes, few dried dates, figs or prunes
Toast with a little low-fat spread

Light Meal
Anchovy and Lentil Pâté, rye crispbreads, carrot and celery sticks
Live low-fat yogurt

Main Meal
Smoked Cod Brandade (see recipe)
Peas or green beans
Fresh fruit

Day 5 – Friday

Breakfast
Custom-made Muesli (see recipe)

Light Meal
Open sandwich or tuna and cucumber sandwich
Fresh fruit

Main Meal
Bean and Leek Bake (see recipe)

Day 6 – Saturday

Breakfast
Fresh Fruit Breakfast Platter: choose from a selection of
  fruits including sliced melon, pineapple, grapefruit,
  banana, pear, apples, strawberries etc. Sprinkle with a
  few pumpkin seeds, sunflower seeds or pistachio nuts

Light Meal
Jacket potato, own choice of filling, mixed salad with lemon
  and olive oil dressing (see recipe)

Main Meal
Avocado Guacamole (see recipe)
Baked fish parcels (see recipe)
Rice
Fruit or live low-fat yogurt

Day 7 – Sunday

Breakfast
Fresh fruit – melon, grapefruit or pineapple
Granary toast, jam with no added sugar

Light Meal
Own choice of soup
Crudités, rye crispbreads
Avocado Guacamole

Main Meal
Bean and Aubergine Pâté, melba toast (see recipe)
Vegetable and Cashew Stir-Fry with egg noodles (see recipe)
Dried Fruit Compote – dried apricots, prunes, pears, apples, peaches etc. cooked in apple juice. Sprinkle with cinnamon and toasted almonds (makes enough for Tuesday breakfast)

Day 8 – Monday

Breakfast
Mushrooms on toast or Muesli

Light Meal
Bean and Aubergine Pâté – crudités and rye crispbreads
Fresh fruit

Main Meal
Tabbouleh (see recipe)
Large green salad

Day 9 – Tuesday

Breakfast
Dried Fruit Compote (from Sunday)

Light Meal
Tabbouleh (from Monday)
Fresh fruit

Main Meal
Sunflower Chicken Stir-Fry (see recipe)

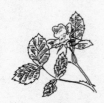

Day 10 – Wednesday

Breakfast
Super Breakfast Shake (see recipe)

Light Meal
Large mixed salad
Live low-fat yogurt

Main Meal
Hummous (see recipe), pitta bread and crudités
Vegetables with Dhal Sauce and Wholegrain Rice
Fresh fruit

Day 11 – Thursday

Breakfast
Scrambled egg on toast or Muesli

Light Meal
Hummous and crudités, rye crispbread or rice cakes
Fresh fruit

Main Meal
Chicken breast baked with garlic, parsley and parmesan
(see recipe)

Day 12 – Friday

Breakfast
Fresh fruit and dried fruit platter

Light Meal
Canned tuna, salmon or mackerel salad sandwich

Main Meal
Pasta Sunshine Salad with low-calorie tomato dressing (see
recipe)
Baked pear or apple, sprinkled with nuts or seeds

Day 13 – Saturday

Breakfast
Custom-made muesli

Light Meal
Smoked Fish Pâté, melba toast (see recipe)

Main Meal
Marinated Tofu with Vegetables and Noodles (see recipe)

Day 14 – Sunday

Breakfast
Dried Fruit Compote or Super Breakfast Shake

Light Meal
Smoked fish pâté in pitta pockets with salad
Fresh fruit

Main Meal
Chilled Gazpacho (see recipe)
Roast Chicken
Vegetables and scrubbed new potatoes
Exotic Fresh Fruit Platter

Recipes

Super Breakfast Shake

Serves 1-2

1 banana
1 egg (optional)
300 ml (½ pint) semi-skimmed milk or soya milk
30 ml (2 tbsp) live natural yogurt
5 ml (1 tsp) honey
5–10 ml (1–2 tsp) unrefined oil

Place all the ingredients into a blender or food processor
and blend into a smooth thick shake. Pour into two large

glasses, sprinkle with nutmeg and serve with wide straws.
   Variation: For a dairy-free shake, omit the milk and yogurt and replace with unsweetened orange, apple or pineapple juice.

Walnut and Mustard Dressing

5 ml (1 level tsp) French mustard, smooth or wholegrain
15 ml (1 tbsp) red wine vinegar
45 ml (3 tbsp) unrefined walnut oil

Whisk together all the ingredients to form a thick smooth dressing. This can be made in larger quantities and stored in an airtight container in the fridge for up to one month.

Lemon and Olive Oil Dressing

2.5 ml (½ level tsp) pale mild mustard
25 ml (1½ tbsp) lemon juice
2.5 ml (½ level tsp) grated lemon rind
60 ml (4 tbsp) unrefined extra virgin olive oil
salt and pepper

Whisk or shake all the ingredients together to form a smooth dressing; the flavour will improve after a few hours. Shake again before serving.

Smoked Cod Brandade

Serves 4

350 g (12 oz) smoked cod
150 ml (¼ pint) semi-skimmed milk
450 g (1lb) potatoes
1–2 garlic cloves, crushed
45–60 ml (3–4 tbsp) extra virgin olive oil or sunflower oil

Place the cod with the milk in a shallow dish and microwave on full power for 5–6 minutes, or poach in a pan until fish flakes easily.
   Scrub the potatoes and boil until tender or cook in the

microwave on full power for 10–12 minutes until tender. Peel and roughly chop the potatoes.

Drain the cod, reserving the liquid, remove skin and bones and place the fish in a blender or food processor, process to a purée. Add the potatoes and process in short bursts to form a fairly coarse purée.

Add the garlic and half the cooking liquid from the fish. Process again, gradually adding the oil through the funnel, add more liquid if necessary to give a soft texture.

Reheat the mixture in the microwave or oven before serving, sprinkled with chopped parsley.

Lunchtime Salad Platter

This is the sort of recipe that changes with the seasons. Adapt and change the vegetables according to what you have. Choose interesting colour, flavour and texture combinations to create a new dish every time.

Line a large serving plate or four individual plates with torn leaves of lettuce, endive and radicchio, sprinkle over bean sprouts or sprouted alfalfa. Make little heaps of different chopped or sliced ingredients all round the plate; try mushrooms, sweetcorn, carrot, courgette, broccoli, cabbage, beetroot, peppers, rice, pasta, etc. Sprinkle over a few olives and almond or cashew nuts plus a few sesame or sunflower seeds.

Sprinkle with 15 ml (1 tbsp) each of unrefined oil and wine vinegar per person or a little dressing.

Anchovy and Lentil Pâté

Serves 4–6

225 g (8 oz) red lentils
1 large onion, chopped
2 garlic cloves, crushed
600 ml (1 pint) vegetable stock
50 g (2 oz) can anchovy fillets
30 ml (2 tbsp) lemon juice
30 ml (2 tbsp) unrefined sesame or walnut oil
25 g (1 oz) fresh wholemeal breadcrumbs

Place the lentils, onion, garlic and stock into a saucepan, bring to the boil, reduce the heat, cover and simmer for about 30 minutes until the lentils are soft and stock is absorbed, add more stock if necessary. The lentils should be soft, losing their shape and the mixture becoming thick and almost dry.

Place the lentil mixture together with the anchovies, lemon juice, oil and breadcrumbs into a food processor or blender, process to give a smooth mixture.

Pour into a serving dish or individual pots and leave to cool. Serve garnished with lemon wedges and chives.

Vegetables with Dhal Sauce

Serves 4

225 g (8 oz) red lentils
600 ml (1 pint) vegetable stock or water
30 ml (2 tbsp) extra virgin olive oil or unrefined sesame
    oil
1 onion, chopped
1 garlic clove, crushed
2.5 cm (1 inch) piece of ginger, peeled and grated
2.5 ml (½ tsp) turmeric
5 ml (1 tsp) cumin
5 ml (1 tsp) coriander
salt and pepper

Place the lentils in a saucepan with the stock, oil, onion, garlic, ginger, spices and salt and pepper, bring to the boil, cover and reduce the heat to a very slow simmer. Cook for about 30 minutes, stirring occasionally and adding more stock if necessary to give a soft but not too thick sauce.

Serve with steamed vegetables and wholegrain rice.

Custom-made Muesli

Here's your chance to make your own personalised muesli containing all your favourites. Make up enough of the dry mixture to give a few servings and save time. (Store in an airtight container in a dark, cool place.)

Base the muesli mixture on 50 per cent oats, then choose a few of the following:

Wheatflakes, oatbran, whole puffed rice
Flaked almonds or hazelnuts
Toasted sunflower or sesame seeds
Raisins, sultanas, apricots, dried apples or dates

Soak a portion of the muesli mixture in unsweetened fruit juice – apple, grape or orange – or skimmed milk or soya milk. Stir in 5 ml (1 tsp) unrefined oil per person and top with fresh fruit – chopped banana, apple, pear, strawberries, etc – plus a spoonful of live low-fat yogurt.

Avocado Guacamole

Serves 4

1 ripe avocado
30 ml (2 tbsp) lemon juice
3 spring onions, finely chopped
2 tomatoes, skinned, deseeded and chopped
1 garlic clove, crushed
few drops of Tabasco sauce
30 ml (2 tbsp) extra virgin olive oil or unrefined sunflower
   or sesame oil
salt and pepper

Halve the avocado, remove the stone and scoop the flesh out into a bowl, sprinkle over half the lemon juice and mash together to form a rough purée. Chop the spring onion and tomatoes finely and add together with the crushed garlic. Whisk together the remaining lemon juice, Tabasco and oil and mix into the avocado mixture. Season to taste. Serve sprinkled with a little paprika.

If a smoother texture is preferred, process all the ingredients together in a blender or food processor until smooth.

Baked Fish Parcels

Serves 4

1 carrot, peeled
1 leek, trimmed
2 celery sticks
4 cod or haddock fillets or cutlets
1 lemon
15 ml (1 level tbsp) sesame seeds
30 ml (2 tbsp) unrefined sesame or sunflower oil

Make four double squares of tinfoil big enough to enclose the fish and vegetables. Cut the carrot, leek and celery into matchsticks and mix together, put half the vegetable mixture into the centre of each piece of foil.

Place the fish on top of the vegetable base and sprinkle the remaining vegetables over the top. Grate a little lemon rind over the top, then squeeze the lemon and mix the juice with an equal quantity of water, divide between the parcels, sprinkling over the fish. Sprinkle over the sesame seeds and drizzle over the oil.

Loosely wrap the foil over the fish to form parcels, place on a baking sheet and cook in the oven, 190°C, (375°F), mark 5 for 20–25 minutes until the fish is tender. Serve with savoury rice.

To microwave: Wrap in greaseproof paper parcels and microwave on full power for 10–12 minutes giving parcels a half turn at half time, to ensure even cooking.

Bean and Aubergine Pâté

Serves 4

1 medium aubergine
2 garlic cloves
400 g (14 oz) can butter beans, drained
45 ml (3 tbsp) live natural yogurt
juice and grated rind of ½ lemon
45 ml (3 level tbsp) chopped fresh herbs
1.25 ml (¼ level tsp) cumin
1.25 ml (¼ level tsp) coriander
30 ml (2 tbsp) extra virgin olive oil

Halve the aubergine, prick with a fork and cook with the whole garlic cloves (unpeeled) in the microwave on full power 5–6 minutes or until soft, or in the oven 200°C (400°F), mark 6 for 30 minutes.

Cool and scoop out the flesh and peel the garlic, place these in a blender or food processor together with the beans, yogurt, lemon, herbs and spices and blend to a smooth purée, dribble in the oil and mix to incorporate. Taste and adjust seasoning and flavourings if necessary.

Vegetable and Cashew Stir-Fry

Serves 4

30 ml (2 tbsp) extra virgin olive oil or sunflower oil
75 g (3 oz) broken cashew nuts
2 carrots, cut into matchsticks
bunch of spring onions, sliced
2 celery sticks, sliced
100 g (4 oz) mange-tout
100 g (4 oz) baby sweetcorn
45 ml (3 tbsp) yellow bean sauce (optional)

Heat 5 ml (1 tsp) of the oil in a wok or large frying pan, cook the cashew nuts until they begin to turn light golden brown.

Add half the remaining oil and all the vegetables and stir-fry for a few minutes, add the remaining oil and stir thoroughly. Add the yellow bean sauce (if using) and heat through.

Serve the stir-fry with egg noodles or brown rice.

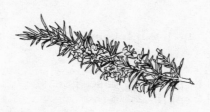

Tabbouleh Cracked Wheat Salad

Serves 4

150 g (5 oz) bulgar cracked wheat
1 vegetable stock cube
½ cucumber, diced
4 tomatoes, chopped
bunch of spring onions, sliced
handful of parsley, chopped
a few mint sprigs, chopped
juice and finely grated rind of 1 lemon
45 ml (3 tbsp) extra virgin olive oil
4 eggs, hard-boiled and quartered
few black olives
45 ml (3 level tbsp) toasted sunflower seeds

Cover the cracked wheat with cold water and leave to soak for up to an hour, drain well and press out all excess moisture. Add the chopped cucumber, tomato, spring onion, parsley and mint.

Mix together the lemon juice, rind and olive oil, pour over the salad and toss together to mix thoroughly. Cover and leave refrigerated for a while before serving to allow flavours to mellow.

Serve garnished with hard-boiled eggs, olives and a sprinkle of sunflower seeds.

Sunflower Chicken Stir-Fry

Serves 4

30 ml (2 tbsp) unrefined sunflower or sesame oil
225 g (8 oz) boneless chicken, cut into strips
30 ml (2 tbsp) light soy sauce
30 ml (2 level tbsp) sunflower seeds
30 ml (2 level tbsp) sesame seeds
3 celery sticks, sliced
175 g (6 oz) bean sprouts

Heat half the oil in a wok or large frying pan, toss in the chicken strips and stir-fry over a medium heat, keeping the chicken moving continuously in the pan for 5 minutes.

Add the remaining oil, soy sauce, sunflower seeds, sesame seeds and vegetables and continue cooking for a further 3 minutes.

Serve with steamed or stir-fried mixed vegetables and egg noodles.

Hummous

Serves 4

1 440g (15½ oz) can chick peas
1 garlic clove, crushed
15–30 ml (1–2 level tbsp) tahini (sesame paste)
30 ml (2 tbsp) lemon juice
salt and paprika
45 ml (3 tbsp) extra virgin olive oil or unrefined walnut or
 hazelnut oil

Drain the chick peas, reserving the liquid, place the chick peas together with the garlic, tahini, lemon juice, oil and seasoning into a blender or food processor. Process to form a smooth thick paste, add a little of the reserved liquid if the mixture is too stiff. Taste and add more tahini, lemon juice or seasoning if necessary. Serve with a little extra oil drizzled over the top, with a sprinkle of paprika and wedges of lemon.

Chicken Breast baked with garlic, parsley and Parmesan

Serves 4

4 chicken breasts, skinned and boned
3–4 garlic cloves, crushed
60 ml (4 tbsp) fresh parsley, chopped
30 ml (2 level tbsp) Parmesan cheese
30–45 ml (2–3 tbsp) extra virgin olive oil

Cut four to five slits diagonally in the top of the chicken fillets and place them in a baking dish with 60–75 ml (4–5 tbsp) water or stock.

Mix together the garlic, parsley, Parmesan and oil and divide the mixture between each chicken breast, rubbing it into the slits well. Cover the dish with foil and bake at 190°C (375°F), mark 5, for 25 minutes or until chicken is cooked through.

Serve with steamed baby vegetables and new potatoes.

Pasta Sunshine Salad

Serves 4

100 g (4 oz) wholewheat pasta shapes
2 carrots, coarsely grated
1 large apple, chopped
1 orange, cut into segments
1 head of chicory, sliced
2 celery sticks, sliced
parsley, chopped
30 ml (2 level tbsp) walnuts, hazelnuts or pine nuts

Cook the pasta until *al dente*, drain and rinse with cold water. When completely cooled, add the grated carrot, apple, orange, chicory, celery and parsley. Pour over the low-calorie tomato dressing (see page 79) and toss to mix well, serve on a bed of salad greens, watercress or alfalfa sprouts, garnish with nuts.

Low-Calorie Tomato Dressing

5 ml (1 level tsp) smooth mild mustard
15 ml (1 tbsp) red wine vinegar
60 ml (4 tbsp) tomato juice
salt and pepper
15–30 ml (1–2 tbsp) unrefined walnut or hazelnut oil

Whisk together the mustard, vinegar, tomato juice and salt and pepper, whisk in the oil and pour immediately over the salad, toss and serve immediately.

Smoked Fish Pâté

Serves 4–6

350 g (12 oz) smoked mackerel or trout
100 g (4 oz) fromage frais or low-fat cream cheese
juice and grated rind of ½ lemon
30 ml (2 tbsp) unrefined safflower or sunflower oil

Skin the fish and remove any bones, place in a blender or
food processor together with the fromage frais, lemon juice
and finely grated rind and the oil and process until smooth
(alternatively pound the fish until smooth in a pestle and
mortar).

Place the mixture in a bowl or individual ramekins, cover
and chill. Serve garnished with a little extra fromage frais
and a sprig of fresh herbs or parsley and a wedge of lemon.

Chilled Gazpacho

Serves 4

600 ml (1 pint) tomato juice
2 slices wholemeal bread
2 garlic cloves, crushed
45 ml (3 tbsp) wine or cider vinegar
30–45 ml (2–3 tbsp) extra virgin olive oil or sunflower oil
½ cucumber
1 red or green pepper, deseeded
4 tomatoes, skinned and deseeded
1 medium onion
salt and pepper

Pour half the tomato juice into a food processor or blender,
pour the remaining half over the bread and leave it to soak.

To the tomato juice, add the garlic, cider vinegar and half
of each vegetable, roughly chopped. Chop the remaining
half very finely ready to add to the soup before serving (or
if a completely smooth texture is preferred, add all the
vegetables). Process until smooth, add the soaked bread
and process again. Add more tomato juice or water, if
necessary, to give the right consistency. Chill before
serving, adding the reserved chopped vegetables.

Personal Favourites

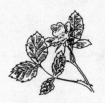

Smoked Salmon Spaghetti Carbonara

Serves 4

225 g (8 oz) wholewheat spaghetti
2 eggs, beaten
30 ml (2 tbsp) unrefined sunflower or safflower oil
100 g (4 oz) smoked salmon pieces, chopped
parsley or fennel

Cook the spaghetti in plenty of boiling salted water until *al dente*, drain and return to the pan.

Whisk the eggs and oil together and stir immediately into the drained spaghetti and toss well. The heat of the spaghetti just begins to cook the eggs. Stir in the smoked salmon and serve on hot plates, sprinkled with fresh herbs.

Bean and Leek Bake

Serves 4

450 g (1 lb) leeks
400 g (14 oz) can butter beans, or fresh broad beans
25 ml (1½ tbsp) unrefined sunflower or safflower oil
25 ml (1½ level tbsp) plain flour
150 ml (¼ pint) semi-skimmed milk or soya milk
700 g (1½ lb) potatoes, thinly sliced

Trim and slice the leeks and cook in a little water until just tender, drain and reserve about 150 ml (¼ pint) of the cooking liquid.

Heat the oil in a small non-stick saucepan, add the flour and cook together for one minute, add the milk and reserved vegetable stock and bring to the boil, stirring together to form a smooth sauce.

Place the cooked leeks and drained beans into the base of an ovenproof dish, pour over the sauce.

Arrange the sliced potatoes over the top, overlapping the layers. Brush with a little extra oil and bake in the oven, at 200°C (400°F), mark 6, for 35–45 minutes or until tender and golden brown.

Marinated Tofu with Vegetables and Noodles

Serves 4

225 g (8 oz) firm tofu
30 ml (2 tbsp) light soy sauce
30 ml (2 tbsp) clear honey
2.5 ml (½ level tsp) Chinese five-spice powder or allspice
30 ml (2 tbsp) unrefined sesame or sunflower oil
1 red pepper, sliced
1 yellow pepper, sliced
100 g (4 oz) mange-tout, green beans or broccoli
100 g (4 oz) baby sweetcorn, fennel or asparagus
225 g (8 oz) egg noodles
15 ml (1 level tbsp) toasted sesame seeds

Cut the tofu into thick slices and halve each slice. Mix together the soy sauce, honey, spice and half the oil and pour the marinade over the tofu, cover and leave for at least an hour.

Steam or stir-fry the vegetables until just tender and cook the egg noodles. Meanwhile heat the remaining oil and sauté the tofu for ½ minute on each side.

Serve the tofu arranged over the egg noodles and vegetables. Sprinkle with toasted sesame seeds.

Hot Potato Salad

Serves 4

700 g (1½ lb) waxy small potatoes (new if possible)
15 ml (1 tbsp) cider vinegar
2.5 ml (½ level tsp) smooth mustard
a pinch of garlic salt
45 ml (3 tbsp) unrefined walnut or hazelnut oil
1 red pepper, chopped
6 spring onions, chopped
200 g (8 oz) can sweetcorn drained
100 g (4 oz) can tuna, optional

Scrub the potatoes and cut into chunks, cook in plenty of boiling salted water until just tender. Meanwhile whisk together the vinegar, mustard, garlic salt and oil to make a smooth dressing.

Drain the cooked potatoes and pour over the dressing, toss quickly then add the chopped pepper, spring onions, sweetcorn and tuna, toss again and serve immediately with a large green salad.

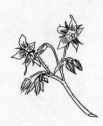

Garlic Dip

Serves 4

10–15 large garlic cloves
175 g (6 oz) fromage frais or low-fat soft cheese
75 g (3 oz) fresh wholemeal breadcrumbs
15–30 ml (1–2 tbsp) unrefined walnut or hazelnut oil
salt and pepper

Place the garlic cloves in a small bowl and just cover with water, microwave on full power for 2–3 minutes until softened (or simmer in a small pan).

Slit and remove skins and place cloves in a blender or food processor together with the soft cheese, breadcrumbs and oil. Season to taste.

Blend all the ingredients to form a fairly smooth soft dip, add a little extra milk if necessary to get a soft consistency.

Serve with crisp raw vegetable crudités and crusty bread.

Herb and Spice Oils

Flavoured oils are easy to make and quickly turn an ordinary oil into a gourmet dressing. Choose a good quality unrefined oil, such as sunflower or virgin olive oil and use two cups of oil to one cup of washed and chopped fresh herbs. Mix well before sealing tightly in a screw-top jar. Store in a cool, dry place for two weeks while the flavours infuse. Once the oil has developed its new flavour, strain off the herbal ingredients and re-bottle the oil, adding a sprig of herbs for decoration. Avoid using plastic containers as these can affect the taste of the oil. Flavoured oils are an excellent base for home-made dressings and can even be drizzled neat over salads. Experiment with your own favourite seasonings, or try these combinations:

- Garlic, basil and crushed peppercorns
- Rosemary, basil and marjoram leaves
- Coriander, fennel and fennel seeds
- Lemon peel and cloves

Garlic Yogurt Dressing

75 ml (5 tbsp) live low-fat natural yogurt
1 garlic clove, crushed
15 ml (1 level tbsp) chopped herbs, parsley, mint etc.
15–30 ml (1–2 tbsp) unrefined sesame or sunflower oil

Whisk all the dressing ingredients together, cover and leave for a while if possible, for flavours to blend. Excellent on winter vegetable salads based on potatoes or cabbage.

Chinese Dressing

15 ml (1 tbsp) cider vinegar
15 ml (1 tbsp) light soy sauce
5 ml (1 tsp) clear honey
2.5 ml (½ level tsp) root ginger, very finely chopped
60 ml (4 tbsp) unrefined oil – sesame, safflower etc.

Mix together the vinegar, soy sauce, honey and ginger, then whisk in the oil to form a thick dressing.

Excellent with crunchy salads using bean sprouts, peppers, mushrooms, baby sweetcorn, mange-tout or carrots.

Foolproof Mayonnaise

2 size 3 egg yolks
5 ml (1 tsp) smooth French mustard
5 ml (1 tsp) honey
30 ml (2 tbs) cider vinegar, wine vinegar or lemon juice
salt and pepper to season
300 ml (½ pint) virgin olive, sunflower or safflower oil

Place the egg yolks, mustard, honey, vinegar and seasoning into a liquidiser or food processor. Blend together until smooth. Keep the machine running and very slowly pour in the oil until it blends into a thick sauce. Refrigerate any unused mayonnaise in an airtight container.

Variations: Add finely chopped fresh herbs, lemon zest, curry powder, tomato puree, horseradish sauce, paprika or Tabasco.

Vitality Salad Dressing

I make this salad dressing every week and always keep a jar of it in the fridge. It has a deliciously light, sweet taste that adds zest to every kind of salad and is bursting with goodness.

45 ml (3 tbsp) virgin olive oil
10 ml (2 tsp) linseed (flax) oil
30 ml (2 tbsp) cider vinegar
5 ml (1 tsp) runny honey
15 ml (1 tbsp) plain, live yogurt
salt and pepper to taste

Tip all the ingredients into a screw-top jar, replace the lid and shake well.

Paddy's Pudding

140 g carton very low-fat, natural live yogurt
   (or very low-fat fromage frais)
150 g (6 oz) ground almonds
10 ml (2 tsp) almond, walnut or hazelnut oil
10 ml (2 tsp) crude blackstrap molasses

This nutritious dessert is very quick to prepare and children love it! Naturally sweet, this recipe provides plenty of iron, calcium and vitamin E. Simply mix all the ingredients together and serve. Also makes a tasty and satisfying breakfast served plain or with a chopped banana.

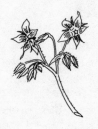

Nutty Biscuit Thins

2 eggs, size 2
150 g (6 oz) soft brown sugar
90 ml (6 tbsp) walnut or hazelnut oil
150 ml (¼ pint) semi-skimmed milk
150 g (6 oz) self-raising flour
30 ml (2 level tbsp) sesame seeds

These light, nutty-flavoured biscuits are delicious with a cup of herb tea and I also serve them with low-fat yogurt.

Pre-heat the oven to 180°C (350°F), mark 4. Mix the eggs with the soft brown sugar to form a thick paste. Add the oil and milk. Fold in the flour and mix until smooth. Grease a baking sheet using a generous amount of olive, sesame or groundnut oil. Drop teaspoonfuls of mixture on to the greased baking tray and sprinkle with sesame seeds. Bake for 10 minutes (5 minutes in a fan-assisted oven) or until the edges turn golden brown. Leave to cool or roll into cigar shapes whilst still warm.

Nut Milks

You can make delicious nut milks by simply whizzing 25 g (1 oz) of nuts with a tumbler of water in the blender. Almonds make a refreshing nut milk and also contain the highest levels of essential fatty acids, calcium and vitamin E. Nut milks can be used in recipes instead of cow's milk or blended with fruit for a satisfying milkshake.

Quick Pasta Sauces

Use these sauces to transform fresh or dried pasta into a culinary extravaganza. Simply blend the ingredients together in a bowl before mixing into cooked, drained pasta. These easy pasta recipes are delicious served with vegetables, chicken or fish dishes, or served on their own as a starter. The sauces can also be used to top grilled or baked fish and will liven up plain jacket potatoes.

Tomato & Herb

30 ml (2 tbs) virgin olive or corn oil
15 ml (1 tbs) cider vinegar
15 ml (1 tbs) tomato purée
5 ml (1 tsp) garlic purée, optional
5 ml (1 tsp) dried oregano or 5 ml (1 tbsp) fresh chopped
  herbs

Parmesan, Garlic & Herb

30 ml (2 tbs) virgin olive or sunflower oil
50 g (2 oz) freshly grated Parmesan cheese
2 cloves garlic, crushed
25 g (1 oz) freshly chopped herbs

Lemon & Olive

30 ml (2 tbs) virgin olive or walnut oil
freshly grated zest from 1 lemon
15 ml (1 tbs) lemon juice
25 g (1 oz) fresh chopped parsley
50 g (2 oz) black olives, quartered

Easy Ways to Add Oils to Your Diet

These ideas will help you easily incorporate unrefined oils into your meals every day. When not using the *Vital Oils Beauty Diet* recipes you can choose one or two of the suggestions each day. Always aim for 15 ml (1 tablespoonful). Worried about the calories? Each 15 ml contains about 125 Kcals, which is roughly equal to 1 oz of cheese, half a pint of beer, 3/4 oz of salted peanuts or two chocolate digestives – but of course far healthier!

Breakfast

Stir a little oil into low-fat yogurt. Mix a spoonful into muesli or porridge.

Milk & Fruit Shakes

Simply whizz up your favourite ingredients in a liquidiser. Base your shake on semi-skimmed milk, soya milk or fruit juice with extra low-fat yogurt or soya yogurt. Add a piece of fresh fruit such as a banana, peach or handful of strawberries. Finish with 15–30 ml (1–2 tablespoonful) of oil per person. Corn, sunflower or safflower are good ones to try.

Dips

These quick and easy crudité dips are based on low-fat soft cheese, fromage frais, Quark or yogurt. Add a little flavouring, choosing from French mustard, tomato purée, Worcestershire sauce, Tabasco, lemon juice and zest, fresh garlic, grated cucumber or freshly chopped herbs. Finish with 15 ml (1 tablespoonful) of oil. Hazelnut or walnut add an excellent flavour. Serve with thin slices of crisp raw vegetables.

Stir-Frys & Steamed Vegetables

Oils are most potent when unheated so stir-fry with the minimum quantity of oil, then just before serving toss in an extra 15 ml (1 tablespoonful) to glaze the vegetables. You can also add oils in this way to steamed vegetables to give them an appetising, glossy shine.

Yogurt, Fruit & Nut Desserts

Make unusual and delicious desserts based on live low-fat yogurt, goat's milk, sheep's milk or soya yogurt. Add chopped or liquidised fresh fruit, finely chopped or ground almonds or hazelnuts plus 15 ml (1 tablespoonful) of oil per person. Choose from unrefined corn, sunflower, sesame or safflower oils.

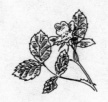

4
It Works!

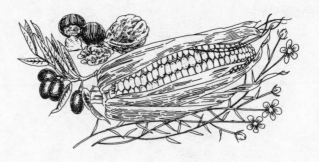

Millions of words are written about healthy eating every year. Sometimes it seems that there are almost more diet books than there are those of us trying to slim. Most regimes promise us the world, but, more often than not, fail to deliver. The best we can expect from many diets is a gnawing hunger and boring range of foods. Remember the egg and grapefruit diet? Or how about a week on watercress milkshakes? The problem with these fad diets is that not only are they nutritionally unsound, but what little weight is lost will pile straight back on the moment we resume our usual eating habits. The secret of the *Vital Oils Beauty Diet*'s success is that it is less a strict weight-loss programme, more a healthy-eating lifestyle. It has been devised to dramatically improve not only our health, but also our looks. And while fighting the flab is important to all of us, its benefits are more far-reaching than weight-loss alone.

In compiling the *Vital Oils Beauty Diet*, I wanted to be sure that the theory behind the regime would be borne out by visible results. The rationale for the eating plan is approved by nutritionists – but how does it stand up in practice? The acid test is a trial by impartial testers, unaware of any of the benefits the eating plan is designed to bring them. So to find out just how well the *Vital Oils Beauty Diet* really works, a nationwide survey was carried out. This involved a random sample of women between the ages of 20 to 50, from the south coast of England to central Scotland. The only criterion for being included in the trial was an interest in taking part. No financial reward or incentive was offered and the panel were unaware that they were testing the *Vital Oils Beauty Diet*. The trials lasted just four weeks. Many thought the length of time too short to see much in the way of results, but the findings were remarkable.

The Evidence

After just four weeks on the *Vital Oils Beauty Diet*, the overwhelming benefits reported were increased energy, vitality and well-being. It was even suggested that the regime should be renamed the Vitality Oils diet! Almost all the panel of testers noticed significant health improvements, with more energy and less symptoms of stress. Well over half the panel of testers found a specific improvement in their appearance within one month, including much better skin and hair condition, and stronger nails. Many of those on the *Vital Oils Beauty Diet* not only felt healthier, they also reported feeling more alert and having greater powers of concentration. In addition to losing weight, most felt better tempered and had fewer common ailments such as colds. This suggests that even in such a short space of time, their immune systems were starting to function more effectively. Even more encouragingly, almost all testers (92 per cent) found the diet easy to follow and said they were able to stick to it without feeling either bored or hungry.

Beauty Benefits

Better Skin
The unrefined oils used in the *Vital Oils Beauty Diet* provide the skin with all of its most important nutrients. These include vitamins A, D and E and, of course, high levels of

essential fatty acids. These nutrients are needed not only to maintain a glowing complexion, but also to help slow the ageing process. Dry, parched skin makes the face look old before its time and the *Vital Oils Beauty Diet* is specifically designed to restore a youthful softness and healthy glow. Despite fears that an oil-enriched diet would cause spots, many testers reported that their complexions were clearer and incidences of spots actually diminished. This is because it is the *type* and *quality* of oil we eat that is a far more important factor than the quantity. Almost all the testers reported some visible improvement to their skin, with benefits ranging from their faces not feeling so dry to their complexions being clearer and fresher looking. Some of the panel noticed that their skin became less sensitive to skincare products and that it didn't feel taut or dry after washing. Not all the beauty benefits were confined to the face though, and one tester remarked that even her cracked and chapped hands improved.

Shinier Hair

Hair growth happens far too slowly for any noticeable results to appear after just one month on the *Vital Oils Beauty Diet* – or so I thought. However, a staggering number of testers reported a visible difference to their hair's condition. In fact, just over half the panel felt that their hair had improved in some way after following the eating plan. This is most likely to be due to a change in the sebaceous secretions that lubricate the scalp and hair strands. These changes can automatically result in naturally glossier, thicker-looking hair. Overall, the testers' hair appeared thicker, shinier and more manageable than before. It also felt softer and silkier to the touch, and needed a little less conditioner after shampooing. Regulating the level of sebum on the scalp also resulted in improved scalp conditions. Several testers found their scalps became less flaky and some cases of dandruff started to clear up. One woman remarked that her recent perm "took on a lot better" as her hair was not so dry. Overall, the *Vital Oils Beauty Diet* is rich in those nutrients needed by hair follicles to function effectively and is a superb long-term plan for strong, healthy hair and for discouraging hair loss.

Stronger Nails

Our nails are even slower to grow than our hair and it takes many months for a new nail to appear from beneath the nail bed. However, nails are made from similar material to our hair and also need many of the same nutrients provided in plentiful supply by the *Vital Oils Beauty Diet*. As a result, 38 per cent of all testers noticed visible improvements after just four weeks. The main comment made by the panel was that their nails appeared to be stronger and did not break as easily. They also seemed to grow faster and were more resistant to splitting. This is probably due to the increased levels of essential fatty acids that help maintain their tensile strength and flexibility.

Health Benefits

Increased Energy

The main aim of the *Vital Oils Beauty Diet* is to promote good looks, better health and encourage well-being. By cutting down on the saturated fats that clog up the system and block the health-giving properties of the essential fatty acids, most *Vital Oil Beauty Diet* testers found their energy levels soared and their health improved. Although aimed at a gradual – and permanent – weight loss, testers found the weight fell away without a struggle. Most testers didn't feel as though they were following a diet at all and many were quite surprised when their weight dropped by a few pounds. Several of the panel commented that they felt more alert and seemed to have greater energy levels than usual. They also reported feeling less tired or sluggish and of feeling unusually well. One tester commented 'I've felt livelier and generally better in myself. I can't believe it – it's great!'

Help for PMS and Stress

The *Vital Oils Beauty Diet* is naturally enriched with the nutrients that play an important part in helping the body cope with hormonal changes, and help regulate the prostaglandin activity that can trigger PMS. Many testers found the time just before their period was easier, and that their stress and concentration levels also improved. This is a typical comment made by one tester: 'My last period was better. I didn't have as much stress leading up to it and noticed a reduced number of painful cramps. I also felt less tired'. Because of its fatty acid balance, other hormonal problems such as symptoms of the menopause can also be expected to improve. Of those testers going through the menopause, several said that their temperamant improved and that they felt less edgy. The *Vital Oils Beauty Diet* also seems to suit working mums and can help career women cope with stressful situations. One tester even reported finding it easier to concentrate on her job than before.

Diet Conclusions

The news is good – the diet works! In fact, it works far better than many sceptics suspected it would. It is clear that we can expect to see a great number of varied health and beauty benefits from just four weeks of following the *Vital Oils Beauty Diet*. The eating plan itself is not hard to follow and the ground rules are reassuringly simple:

- Eat much less saturated fat
- Use only pure, unrefined cooking oils
- Include 15 ml (1 tablespoonful) of uncooked oil in your meals each day.

While the benefits of healthy eating can be clearly seen after a few weeks, the advantages for long-term good health can only be expected to continue if you keep up the good work. Don't be tempted to slip back into old habits and unhealthy eating patterns. Yes, the unrefined oils do cost a little more, but you will use less of them as the recipes don't involve large quantities. Besides, it is a very small price to pay for the huge health and beauty potential. I am not going to claim that this eating plan will cure all known diseases or improve your sex life – but what it can do is give your body the best possible chance of boosting energy levels, increase its resistance to disease and even help it fight serious disorders such as heart disease and arthritis. And as the research has shown, the *Vital Oils Beauty Diet* not only restores your vitality, but will leave you feeling good and looking even better.

5

Applying Oils For Beauty

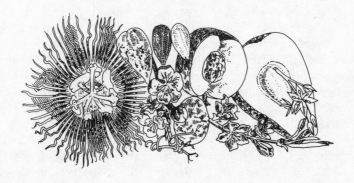

There is no doubt that eating the right type of oils can improve our health and vitality, but natural plant oils can have a dramatic effect on the skin too. Their benefits are twofold. Firstly, eating oils in our diet or by swallowing them in the form of supplements we can dramatically improve our complexion and delay the signs of ageing. Secondly, by applying oils directly to the skin we provide it with many of the nutrients needed to keep it supple and strong. Oils are such effective moisturisers that they are the key ingredient in most rejuvenating and anti-ageing skin treatments. Some plant oils, such as wheatgerm, are a wonderfully rich source of vitamin E which neutralise the free-radicals that cause cell damage. Free-radicals attack the collagen and elastin protein fibres that support the skin, making it appear saggy and slack. But by using oils that are rich in essential fatty acids and vitamin E – both internally and externally – we're able fight the war on wrinkles from two powerful fronts.

Although natural oils are important ingredients in sophisticated skincreams, their use in beauty treatments is nothing new. Oils have been highly prized for centuries for their therapeutic skincare effects and one of the earliest recorded uses of oil on the skin is in the New Testament. 'Mary took a pound of costly spikenard and anointed the feet of Jesus', John 12:3. This simple gesture was, in fact, the height of extravagance as spikenard was an extremely expensive, aromatic oil from the remote valleys of the Himalayas. It was extracted from the tiny roots of the fragile spikenard plant, and this amount would have cost the average labourer an entire year's wages. Another ancient oil found in the Bible is cassia oil, produced from cinnamon trees. Cassia oil is extracted from cinnamon bark and was mixed with olive oil which was in plentiful supply around Palestine. The resulting blend was used after bathing to keep the skin soft, smooth and sweetly scented.

In Ancient Egypt, Queen Cleopatra was famed for the amount of time she spent beautifying herself and her narcissistic regime included face masks and massage lotions made from these nourishing seeds. An Egyptian stone carving at Deir-el-Bahari shows a woman applying oil to her hair and in the temple of Hatshepsut at Thebes there are paintings of high-ranking Egyptian women having their shoulders massaged with aromatic oils. This treatment has been revived this century and renamed aromatherapy, and it remains a highly effective way of conditioning the skin.

Pure, unrefined oils have certainly withstood the test of time and scientists have yet to improve on their ability to protect and repair the skin. Despite many millions of pounds spent on research and development by the cosmetic industry each year, these natural oils remain our most valuable and versatile skincare assets.

Almond Oil (Prunus amygdalus)

Almond oil is another health and beauty oil that can be traced back for centuries. There are two types of almond tree – the bitter almond that produces white blossom and the sweet almond that produces pink blossom. The type of oil used for beauty preparations is warm-pressed from sweet almond kernels and is sometimes referred to as 'sweet almond oil'. The earliest use of almond oil in this country was during the Roman occupation, when it was first introduced to Britain. It was obviously a great success as almond oil continued to be an important element of skincare throughout medieval times. In 1372, the Queen of France is recorded as ordering 227 kilos (500 lb) of almonds with the sole purpose of extracting their oil for her face creams. Later, Napoleon's wife Josephine ran up equally extravagant bills for 'crème amande' which she used as a hand cream and moisturiser. Almond oil was a favourite beautifier throughout Europe, and in Britain the 16th-century herbalist John Gerard wrote 'oil of almonds makes smoothe thye hands and face of delicate persons and cleanseth the skin from spots and pimples.' Almond oil was also the base for the famous hair tonic, Macassar oil, which consisted of almond oil scented with cassia extracts.

Almond oil is a useful source of vitamin D and is traditionally associated with strong, healthy nails. One of the simplest nail treatments is to warm a few drops of almond oil in the palms of your hands before massaging it around the base of the nail and cuticles. The cosmetics industry is still a major purchaser of almond oil. It is added to a great number of modern, emollient formulae, from hair conditioners to hand creams. Almond oil is available from health food stores and chemists and is a useful ingredient for home-made skincare. Ground almonds also contain useful amounts of the oil and are good for adding to skin scrubs. The action of rubbing the granules over the skin releases the natural oil and leaves the skin smooth and moisturised.

Apricot Oil (Prunus armeniaca)

Apricot oil is similar in structure to peachnut oil, except that it is higher in polyunsaturates. However, for beauty purposes, it has the same light texture and can be used in exactly the same way. The apricot tree is small and twiggy with an abundance of white flowers tinged with red that appear at the begining of spring. Its botanical name, *Prunus armeniaca*, comes from the Latin for plum and it is a member of the plum family. Apricot trees flourish in temperate climates and were first noted in Armenia and China. While the apricot fruits are rich in beta carotene, the vegetable precursor to vitamin A, the oil comes from the seed kernel and contains only traces of vitamins. However, apricot oil does contain useful levels of essential fatty acids. It also has a wonderfully light texture making it very easily absorbed into the skin.

Avocado Oil (Persea americana)

Avocado oil is a traditional beauty oil which was used by the tribeswomen of Mexico and Arizona. The oil comes from the flesh of the avocado and was one of the easiest vegetable oils for early civilisations to extract. The avocado tree was first found growing in South American swamp-lands and still carries the nickname 'alligator pear'. It is a distant relative of the magnolia and bay laurel and grows in California, Mexico, Florida and Mediterranean countries. The Aztecs were the first fans of this fruit and claimed it was an aphrodisiac. Other cultures used avocado oil for more medicinal purposes and in the Philippines it was sold as a cure for conditions as diverse as toothache and dysentery. In the early 16th century the Franciscan priest Toribio de Montolinia recorded its use in Mexico and wrote 'Among the fruits found in the mountains is one they call "ahuacatl", which hangs on the tree and looks like a large pear. The fruit is so wholesome that it is served to the sick. Water prepared from the broad, green leaf is good as a remedy for the legs and even better for the face.' Since then, avocado oil has continued to be acclaimed for its skincare properties and to be an important ingredient for the cosmetic industry.

Although we mostly use avocado in savoury recipes, technically it is a fruit because it contains a stone. Avocados are highly nutritious, being rich in protein, lecithin and vitamins A, B and D. Despite their high oil content, avocados do not contain any cholesterol, but they do have high levels of beneficial linoleic acid, the parent of GLA. The oil comes from the exceptionally oily flesh which consists of up to 30 per cent pure oil – a figure rivalled only by the olive and palm fruit. Crude avocado oil is produced by mechanical pressing on hydraulic presses, followed by centrifugal extraction. It is not usually extracted using solvents. Oil may also be extracted from the stone, although this is not used by the beauty industry. The oil from the stone contains a condensed flavanol called biscatechin which is reported to have an anti-tumour effect in cases of skin cancer in rats and mice. However, some reports state that the oil from the stone is highly poisonous and more research is needed into its exact properties. By contrast, oil from the flesh of the avocado is highly nutritious and rich in many nutrients including vitamins A and D, and the mineral potassium. Although the oil is monounsaturated, it is not as stable as olive oil at high temperatures and so not as suitable for cooking. In its crude state, avocado oil contains large amounts of chlorophyll that colour it a dazzling shade of emerald green. Crude avocado oil is mainly bought by toiletry manufacturers who add it to a wide range of products including cleansing cream, moisturiser, hair conditioner, bath oil, suntan lotion, foundation and lipstick. Its mild, nutty flavour also appeals to the food industry, although it quickly turns rancid if exposed to the air or daylight. This means that almost all edible avocado oil goes through extensive refining processes that reduce it to a pale shade of yellow. One way to protect avocado oil from spoilage is to pack it into individual capsules and this is a very convenient way of taking the oil.

Avocado oil is a time-tested skin soother and softener, but scientists are only begining to realise its full skincare potential. Research carried out in America has revealed that avocado oil not only smoothes the surface of the skin but can also slip through and penetrate its upper layers. Clinical trials have shown avocado oil to be more easily absorbed by the skin than other well-known cosmetic oils such as olive and sweet almond. By carrying its vital vitamins and essential fatty acids below the surface of the skin, avocado oil could play an important part in delaying skin degeneration and slowing the signs of ageing.

Many vegetable oils are natural sunscreens – and again avocado beats the other beauty oils in its ability to block out the sun's rays. Studies show that the oils most able to block the sun's harmful rays are (in order) avocado, sweet almond, sesame, safflower, coconut and olive. The sun is the skin's number-one enemy for encouraging fine lines and wrinkles. It is also the cause of the more worrying increase in the level of skin cancers. As a result, sunscreen technology has become one of the most important areas of cosmetic research. However, many of the chemical compounds used such as PABA (para-aminobenzoic acid) are common skin irritants. Avocado oil is highly compatible with all but the most sensitive skin types, and while research into its exact scientific properties goes on, it could lead to avocado oil becoming our most valuable cosmetic ingredient yet.

Castor Oil (Ricinus communis)

Castor oil is a natural oil that is better known for its powers as a laxative than for its effect on the skin. However, it is used in protective hair and skincare products. Castor oil comes from the castor plant, which is native to West Africa and the Mediterranean countries. It is a small, thorny shrub with blue-green leaves and tiny pink flowers that cluster along its spiky stems. An attractive shrub, the castor oil plant also makes a decorative indoor plant. The castor beans lurk beneath the profusion of flowers and contain its many hundreds of glossy brown seeds. These seeds contain a poisonous resin that is activated by heat, and so the oil must be cold-pressed. Because of this resin, castor oil has a limited use in the world of health and beauty, but it is a useful waterproofing agent. Its lubricating and water-repelling properties are most useful for hair shiners and babies' nappy rash creams. Castor oil is also found in some hair lacquers and can be blended with emollients such as lanolin to make barrier creams. Despite its unpleasant smell, castor oil rarely causes an allergic reaction, and is used in many ointments. It also has the ability to clear red eyes and is even used in eye drops.

The castor oil plant features in herbal medicine as a laxative and is now widely grown for its oil which is used as a commercial lubricant. Many old wives' tales surround the purgative effects of castor oil and it is reputed to have the ability to induce labour. As a last resort measure for overdue babies, some midwives still suggest knocking back half a glass of castor oil mixed with orange juice (to make it slightly more palatable). However, there is little evidence that this works and it is more likely to leave the imbiber severely dehydrated.

Coconut Oil (Cocos nucifera)

South Sea islanders are renowned for glossy tresses and smooth, sunkissed skin – despite the fiercely drying effects of the sun. Their secret is coconut oil, which is extracted from the dried flesh of the coconut. This dried flesh is called copra and it contains an extraordinary amount of oil, about 65 per cent on average. Coconuts are the fruits of the hardy palm tree that thrives on dry, sandy soils. The tree is a botanical giant, growing over 15 metres (50 feet) high with leaves that measure up to 1.82 metres (6 feet) long. The fragrant white coconut flowers are closely followed by huge fruit that weigh over one kilo (2.2 lb) and are enclosed in a hard protective shell. Coconut oil is an important ingredient in the beauty business and is mainly used in soaps and natural cleansers. It has a low-lathering cleansing action and is often added to shampoos and the more expensive detergents. Coconut oil can also be used by itself and the Tagai women of the Philippine Islands comb it through their long black hair to give it a high-gloss shine. They also mix coconut oil with sandalwood oil to make a blend called 'monoi' which helps their skin stay soft and sweet-smelling in the heat. Coconut palms grow on tropical coasts and the principal oil-producing countries are the Philippines, Malaysia, Sri Lanka and Indonesia.

Evening Primrose Oil (Oenothera biennis)

The latest natural oil to be used in skincare is evening primrose oil. Not only does this oil have dramatic effects on the skin when swallowed, it can also improve the skin's appearance when applied directly to the surface. One of the signs that the body is having problems converting linoleic acid into GLA is a dry, flaky complexion. This can be for many reasons. It may be that the body isn't getting sufficient supplies from the diet, or that the conversion process is being hindered by viral infection, alcohol, smoking or hereditary factors. While a daily internal dose of evening primrose oil can significantly improve the look and feel of dry skin, the capsules can also be pierced and the contents rubbed into the skin. The GLA in the evening primrose oil will be absorbed by the uppermost layers of skin cells and will help prevent vital moisture loss. Because it is a quite sticky, concentrated oil it is easiest to use when blended with another lighter oil, such as grapeseed or safflower. This mixture then forms a protective layer on the epidermis and keeps the complexion supple and strong. The mixture will keep for about a month if stored in a cool, dark place, and can be used instead of expensive skin creams or body lotions. The capacity of evening primrose oil to care for the skin has meant that an increasing number of skincare ranges use it. However, because the oil is an expensive ingredient and has a limited shelf life, few creams contain significant quantities. To get the maximum benefit from the oil, I prefer to add the fresh contents of a capsule to a small jar of moisturiser, and use this within a few weeks before making more.

Jojoba Oil (Simmondsia chinensis)

Jojoba oil (pronounced ho-ho-ba) comes from the jojoba shrub in South America and is a valuable newcomer to the cosmetics industry. The jojoba plant is a hardy evergreen that grows 0.6–1.82 metres (2–6 feet) tall with small dark brown beans. The jojoba plant is one of the few that thrive in arid, desert regions, and will withstand the fierce climatic conditions of strong winds, fierce heat and prolonged drought. The oil is extracted from the beans, and technically speaking, it is more of a wax than an oil as it is solid at room temperature. Jojoba is another of mother nature's beauty assets, and has a long-standing traditional use by the American Indians in Mexico and Arizona where the beans grow wild. Jojoba oil is valuable because it requires little or no refining, and has several specific skincare properties. Its chemical composition is close to the skin's own oil, sebum, making it good for all skin types. Because of its natural affinity with the skin, jojoba oil is especially good for sensitive complexions, or oily and acne skin conditions that require delicate treatment. When massaged into the skin, jojoba oil combines with sebum and gently unclogs pores to free embedded dirt and grime. Although jojoba oil is naturally solid, it melts at body temperature. This means that it produces a firm texture for skin creams, yet swiftly melts when rubbed on the skin. In addition, jojoba oil has unusual anti-bacterial properties that resist spoilage and rancidity. This means that jojoba oil has a very long shelf life, and can be left unopened with less fear of rancidity than the other natural oils.

Jojoba oil is a vegetable alternative to the oil of the great sperm whale and its use was developed during the 1970s when the whale became listed as an endangered species. Technically, spermaceti is neither an oil nor a fat, but a waxy substance from the head of the sperm whale. This gruesome extract was a common ingredient in many mass-market moisturisers as it does have superb skin-softening properties. It was also used to thicken skin creams and give them a glossy shine. Both cheap and highly emollient, spermaceti has featured in skincare since 1785. Fortunately, spermaceti and other whale imports are now banned in Europe, America and most other enlightened nations. Jojoba oil has the advantage of being a cheap, cruelty-free alternative, and is thankfully reducing the worldwide demand for whale oil. To ensure that there are sufficient supplies of jojoba oil to satisfy the increased demand, an extensive planting programme is being carried out in developing countries of the Third World. While these crops have yet to come to fruition, they should at least secure the future of some of the world's poorest people – and the great sperm whale.

Olive Oil (Olea europea)

Olive oil is mankind's original skin soother and was the very first oil used in beauty treatments. As we have already seen in Chapter Two, its health benefits are far-ranging, but it plays an important part in caring for the skin too. The cosmetic benefits of olive oil have been recognised for thousands of years, and it was originally used by the Ancient Greeks and Egyptians for body massage. A useful source of vitamin E, olive oil is wonderfully soothing and will instantly take the heat out of sore, inflamed skin. Hippocrates prescribed olive oil for sunburn, and it is still a useful after-sun soother. Olive oil has a rich, slightly sticky texture and can be combined with lighter oils, such as grapeseed, for massage blends. Its power as an emollient is recognised by the medical profession and purified olive oil is used in hospitals to treat chapped and scaly skin conditions. My own daughter was born two weeks late and with severely dehydrated skin. The first thing I was given was olive oil to massage her with and within days her skin was as smooth and soft as a baby's should be! As well as nourishing the skin, olive oil also makes a useful hair conditioner as it increases the tensile strength of the hair shafts. Its rich texture is especially suited to giving body and shine to slightly coarse, thick hair. A few drops combed through the ends of very dry hair will also tame frizzy, fly-away ends.

Passionflower Oil (Passiflora incarnata)

The passionflower is a herbaceous perennial plant native to South America and later cultivated all over the Mediterranean. It was introduced to Britain from Brazil in the 17th century and grows in gardens on the south coast of England or under glass elsewhere in Britain. The passion-flower is a fast-climbing plant and likes to grow along sunny south-facing walls and trellises. The passionflower takes its name from the stunning purple-tinged yellow or pink flowers that are said to illustrate the crucifixion, or passion, of Christ. The flowers have a group of central filaments or 'corona' that resemble the crown of thorns, while the stigmata is in the shape of the cross with the stamens representing the nails. The flowers give way to large orange berries called passion fruit, which are roughly the size and shape of a small apple. Inside the passion fruit's hard outer casing is a soft yellow pulp that contains a mass of blackened seeds. Passionflower oil is warm-pressed from these seeds and is not usually extracted with solvents. It contains a high percentage of linoleic acid, the parent of GLA. Passionflower oil is polyunsaturated and it is produced in capsule form combined with evening primrose oil to promote and maintain skin elasticity.

The leaves and flowering tops of the passionflower have very different qualities from the oil and are used by herbalists as anti-spasmodics and relaxants. These sedative properties were first noticed in the late 19th century by American physicians who used passiflora extract in the field of neurology. Passiflora extract is a narcotic, with a similar chemical composition to morphine. The extract is often combined with other calming herbs such as scullcap, hawthorn and valerian to make powerful sedative brews. Passiflora extract is the main ingredient in a German sleeping pill called Vita-Dor, which is commonly prescribed for treating insomnia. And in Rumania, a patent was recently issued for a sedative chewing gum that also contains passiflora extract. Studies have identified the alkaloid 'maltol' as being the active principle present that causes the sedative action. The French medical herbalist Leclerc also uses passiflora extract to treat nervous disorders appearing at the time of the menopause. Passiflora extract has also been used to successfully treat bronchitis and asthma, and as a topical treatment for burns. Herbal compresses containing the extract appear to reduce inflammation. However, passionflower oil itself does not have any sedating or anti-inflammatory properties and is principally used in beauty treatments for its fine texture and, when in its raw state, its high levels of essential fatty acids.

Peachnut Oil (Prunus persica)

Peachnut oil originates from China and is another ancient oil reputed to have been brought to Britain by the Romans. The oil comes from the peach kernels of the *Prunus persica* tree, which is distinguished in springtime by its bright pink flowers. The peach tree likes a limey soil with plenty of strong sunshine in the summer months and cold, dry winters. If the climatic conditions are right, the peach tree can happily thrive for several hundred years. Peaches need plenty of sunshine to ripen and are ready for picking towards the end of the summer. The fruits are then sliced open prior to canning, while the kernels are cold-pressed to yield the oil.

Peachnut oil is a pale golden colour and has a light, sweet smell. When used on the skin it supposedly encourages the body to secrete its own natural oils, making it a natural favourite for facial massage. Peachnut oil is high in both mono- and polyunsaturates and can be taken as a supplement to promote hair texture and shine. It also contains useful levels of essential fatty acids and vitamin E, making it a useful supplement to encourage skin suppleness and elasticity. Peachnut oil is increasingly available in its natural, unrefined state and is a useful ingredient for home-made skincare and massage blends.

Sesame Oil (Sesamum indicum)

The sesame plant is another native of southern Asia and the Mediterranean and also has a long association with the world of beauty. The plant itself is a leafy shrub scattered with pinkish white flowers. It requires several months of constant, hot sunshine to ripen the seedpods that contain its seeds. Sesame oil is extracted from these seeds, which can contain up to 60 per cent pure oil. Sesame oil has been used for thousands of years in beauty treatments and was widely used by the Ancient Egyptians, Greeks and Romans. It has a fine, light texture and almost no smell, making it an ideal base for massage oils. Sesame oil is also a useful sunfilter and screens out up to 30 per cent of the sun's harmful rays. This compares well with other vegetable oils that screen out, on average, 20 per cent of the sun's rays. Sesame oil is still used as a natural moisturiser by Mediterranean women as it nourishes the skin whilst offering a degree of protection against burning. It is also a common component of modern suntan oils. Sesame oil is a monounsaturated oil and like olive oil, is less likely to turn rancid in the heat.

Wheatgerm Oil (Triticum vulgare)

Wheatgerm oil is another natural oil with a long and noble history. Traces of the oil have been found in Egyptian tombs dating back to 2000 BC and in prehistoric lake dwellings in Switzerland. Wheat is one of the world's most important foods, and is the largest crop grown in Britain today. Wheatgerm oil is extracted by warm-pressing or solvent expression from the 'germ' of wheat. It is extremely rich and nourishing, and is one of our richest sources of vitamin E (190 mg per 100 g) and essential fatty acids. Because of its vitamin E content, wheatgerm oil is a natural antioxidant and is well protected from the elements that usually break down vegetable oils, such as light and heat. Wheatgerm oil is too rich and sticky to use on its own, but it is very useful when added in small amounts to other oils to boost their nutritional content and guard against rancidity. Wheatgerm oil is used in natural beauty preparations to treat dry, mature skin and is a versatile ingredient for home-made skincare. Wheatgerm husks are also a good source of the B complex vitamins and vitamin E, and can be included in a number of concoctions for the skin. One of the simplest and most nourishing face packs consists of wheatgerm and plain yogurt mixed together in equal quantities to form a rich paste.

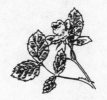

6

The Essential Oils

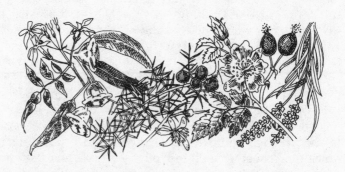

Essential oils are highly aromatic natural extracts which have been described as the 'spirit' or 'soul' of a plant. They are contained in tiny oil glands or sacs in plants and each root, leaf or flower has its own unique fragrance. Each essential oil has unique therapeutic properties and they are the most versatile of all beauty oils. There are about 300 different types of these aromatic essences, each extracted from the flowers, leaves, stalks, seeds, roots or rind of a plant. The use of essential oils has increased dramatically in recent years and now every health food shop, department store and chemist seems to stock a selection.

However, their use in health and beauty treatments is nothing new and they have been known to holistic practitioners for literally thousands of years. One of the first recorded uses of essential oils was by an Egyptian called Imhotep, who used them in massage treatments and was later deified as a god of medicine and healing. The use of essential oils in the bath is also long established and 2500 years ago Hippocrates wrote that he found aromatic baths useful in the treatment of feminine disorders. All essential oils are antiseptic and as far back as 1800 BC the Babylonians used myrrh, cypress and cedarwood oils to ward off infections. The Romans added drops of sweet-smelling essential oils to their baths, and the father of medicine, Hippocrates, stated that 'the way to good health is to take an aromatic bath and fragrant massage every day'. About 1000 years ago the use of essential oils as medicines started to decline, although they have continued to crop up from time to time throughout history. During the 13th century, France became an important perfume centre and was the world's leading producer of essential oils. Even though diseases such as yellow fever were rife at the time, the perfume workers were rarely affected, and it is thought that the antiseptic qualities of the oils protected them. Studies have since shown that the micro-organisms responsible for yellow fever are easily killed by essential oils. French essential oil production mainly centred around Grasse, situated high in the hills in the south of France. Here the abundant sunshine and well-drained soil suits the fields of exotic flowers needed to make fine fragrances. Grasse was originally a tannery centre, and the perfumers sold their wares to the leather-workers who made fragranced gloves. In the 18th century bathing was deemed to be unhealthy and so no-one took much notice of personal hygiene. As a result, fragranced gloves were popular amongst the gentry to mask the smell of body odour. Nowadays essential oils are produced all over the world, but Grasse still has a reputation for producing some of the finest floral extracts.

The French Connection

Although the therapeutic powers of essential oils have been known for thousands of years, it was not until 1937 that they were scientifically analysed. The man credited with cataloging their medicinal properties was the French cosmetic scientist, René-Maurice Gattefossé, who coined the term 'aromatherapy'. Gattefossé first realised the healing potential of these oils after he badly burnt his hand during a laboratory experiment. To relieve the pain he plunged it into the nearest vat of liquid, which just happened to be lavender oil. Gattefossé was amazed at how quickly the oil soothed his inflamed skin and helped it to heal. Another Frenchman convinced of the powers of essential oils was the Parisian army surgeon, Jean Valnet. During the the Second World War, Dr Valnet used essential oils as antiseptics to treat war wounds. He also noticed that the troops who slept rough in the dense pine forests suffered from fewer respiratory infections. Recognising that the aroma from the pine trees was the active ingredient, Dr Valnet used essential oils as the focus of his work. When the war ended, Dr Valnet wrote *Aromathérapie*, published in 1964, which is now published in English and has become the aromatherapist's bible. The French are far more accepting of the powers and therapeutic properties of essential oils, and there are several medical schools that include the study of essential oils as part of their curriculum. A form of herbal medicine called phytotherapy is widely practised across Europe today and this also features the use of essential oils.

Extracting Essential Oils

Although they are termed 'essential' these highly concentrated extracts should not be confused with the edible vegetable and fish oils that contain essential fatty acids and vitamins. Essential oils are the odorous, volatile extracts of a single plant and consist of carbon, hydrogen and oxygen atoms. They are chemically quite distinct from edible fats and oils, and should not be consumed. Essential oils can come from any part of a plant and their 'volatility' simply means that they will evaporate if left open to the air. Different oils can be extracted from different parts of the same species, such as the orange tree, whose flowers yield neroli oil; leaves and twigs produce petitgrain oil; and fruit rind produces bitter orange oil.

Enfleurage

The oldest method of extracting essential oil is enfleurage, and this is still one of the best methods of obtaining the oil from fragile flower heads such as jasmine. Within hours of picking, the flowers are placed on sheets of glass that have been covered with purified animal fat or beeswax. As the oil from the flowers soaks into the fat, so more layers of petals are added until the fat is completely saturated with essential oil. This method of extraction particularly suits jasmine blossoms which continue to release their aroma for 24 hours after picking. The fragrant mulch produced at this stage is called a 'pomade' and was used in its raw state as a gentleman's hair dressing. To release the oil, the pomade is dissolved in alcohol and the fat sinks to the bottom of the container. The mixture is then heated so that the alcohol evaporates, leaving the pure essential oil behind. The enfleurage extraction process is still carried out by hand, and is much more time-consuming than other more mechanised methods. Even collecting the raw materials, is highly labour-intensive. It's estimated that it takes a staggering 8 million jasmine flowers to produce a single kilo of pure essential oil. Not surprisingly, jasmine is one of the world's most expensive fragrant essences.

Distillation

These days, however, most essential oils are extracted by distillation. This method was invented in the 11th century by the Arabian herbalist Avicenna. During an alchemy experiment using rose petals, Avicenna discovered that if the flowers were placed in a flask and heated, the vapour could be collected in another flask. Avicenna identified this fragranced vapour as rosewater and the substance floating on its surface as pure rose oil. The modern process of distillation involves combining the aromatic part of the plant with boiling water or steam. The vapour then travels along a series of glass tubes that form a condenser. The essential oil droplets are siphoned off through a narrow-necked container, and the remaining water collected in a container below. The essential oil may then be filtered before bottling. Distillation is by far the most common extraction method and works well for most essential oils, including the exquisite rose otto.

Solvent Extraction

Technically speaking, the process of solvent extraction yields 'absolutes' and not pure essential oils. It is a method primarily used by the perfume industry to release the fragrance from flowers and is a cheaper alternative to distillation. Solvent extraction is a highly mechanised procedure and many aromatherapists feel that the end product is devitalised and lacking in therapeutic properties. Solvent extraction begins by mixing flower petals together with a solvent such as hexane in huge metal vats. These are then stirred with rotating paddles that encourage the petals to release their oils. After several hours, the petals are strained off, leaving a mixture of solvent and perfumed 'absolute' behind. To retrieve the absolute, the mixture is heated so that the solvent evaporates away. Rose, orange blossom and mimosa are the most common absolutes produced by solvent extraction. All are labour-intensive as the blooms must be picked by hand. And it takes approximately 6000 kilos (15,230 lb) of petals to produce a single kilo (2.2 lb) of rose absolute.

Expression

Citrus oils such as lemon and mandarin are more easily, and cheaply, available and are extracted by a process called expression. In the old days, the rinds of the fruits were squeezed by hand to extract the oil from the multitude of tiny glands visible in the peel. Nowadays the process is highly mechanised and the fruit is first crushed before being placed in a centrifugal extractor. This rotates at high speed to spin out the droplets of essential oils.

How to Use Essential Oils

Essential oils are highly versatile healers and can be used in many different ways. They can be diluted for face and body massage, added to a bath, burnt to give off an aroma, inhaled in hot water, used in a compress or even applied neat in small quantities on burns and scars. Essential oils provide the basis of aromatherapy, which literally means 'treatment with aromas'. The woman credited with bringing aromatherapy within reach of the public was Madame Marguerite Maury. This French biochemist with an interest in beauty therapy worked with Dr Jean Valnet and is responsible for bringing aromatherapy as we know it to Britain. Madame Maury recognised the value of applying oils to the skin using specific massage techniques and developed the holistic principles behind aromatherapy today. Based at her London clinic she trained not only beauty therapists but also nurses, physiotherapists, medical herbalists and doctors seeking alternatives to conventional drug treatments. Aromatherapists who trained under Madame Maury include Micheline Arcier and Daniele Ryman. These women are now the doyennes of the aromatherapy world and have their own clinics, training facilities and ranges of essential oils. Many of the newer aromatherapy organisations are also well respected. Aromatherapy Associates are held in high regard, and have one of the most attractive and holistic clinics I've come across. Although all those mentioned are based in London, there are now accredited aromatherapists nationwide. Further details on how to find an aromatherapist or aromatherapy training can be found at the end of this book.

There are two parts to aromatherapy, the first is the smell of the oil and the second is the action it has on the body. Our sense of smell is the most powerful of all our senses and has a dramatic effect on the way we feel. It is controlled by the olfactory organ situated above the nose, just below the base of our brain. The olfactory organ is covered with a thin sheet of membrane housing approximately 800 million nerve endings. These nerve endings are there solely to detect smells and are so tiny that they can barely be seen under a powerful electron microscope. Whenever we catch a whiff of something, our olfactory nerves send scent messages to the limbic system in the brain. This is responsible for controlling our moods and emotions and explains why the aromas from essential oils can have such a profound effect on the way we feel. The limbic system is capable of remembering many millions of different smells and nothing evokes a memory faster than a specific smell.

Because they are so powerful, essential oils are usually diluted before they're used on the skin, and a few drops in a spoonful of vegetable oil will be enough to cover the entire body. Essential oils have a very small molecular structure which enables them to slip through the network of surface skin cells and end up in the bloodstream. Experiments using essential oils show that within half an hour of being applied to the skin, traces of essential oil appear in the urine. We also know that essential oils are rapidly excreted from the body and so there is little danger of overdose. However, essential oils must not be taken internally unless under the strict guidance of a qualified aromatherapist or doctor, as they can burn the delicate mucus membranes that line the mouth, throat and stomach.

Massage Oils

Essential oils do not dissolve in water but do dissolve in oil, so need mixing with a 'carrier' oil to disperse them on the skin. There are two steps to making a massage oil. The first is to choose which kind of carrier oil will make the best base for your blend. Grapeseed oil has a fine, light texture and is popular with aromatherapists for body massage oils. Sunflower and safflower oils are also light textured, while corn oils are a little too sticky and have a slight smell. For facial massage I prefer using blends of jojoba, avocado, peachnut, apricot kernel and almond oils. These are more expensive carrier oils, but they only need to be used in small quantities as a little goes a very long way. I also add a few drops of wheatgerm oil to my massage blends. Wheatgerm is rich in vitamin E and an excellent natural antioxidant, and will protect the oils from rancidity. All massage oils should be made with unrefined oils where possible as these oils still retain their important skin-nourishing nutrients. The reason I don't ever use baby oil is that it is a mineral oil and a processed by-product of the petroleum industry. Being a highly refined product, baby oil lacks natural, skin-nourishing nutrients. Most baby oils also contain synthetic perfumes, and I prefer to use pure essential oils that have their own therapeutic benefits.

The Carrier Oils

Choose from the following base oils for making your own massage blends. These oils are safe for all skin types, but it is advisable to patch test the carrier oils first before making the blend. A very few people with highly sensitive complexions can develop an allergic reaction even to natural oils, so it is worth testing each one you use on a small area of skin first. When preparing oils for the face, only use pure, top quality oils.

Almond Oil

A slightly sticky oil which is especially suited to body massage blends. Good for most skin types, especially dry, easily irritated complexions. Containing vitamins and minerals, almond oil can help relieve itch and swelling. Use on its own or blend with grapeseed, jojoba or sunflower oils.

Apricot Kernel Oil

The light texture of this oil is especially suitable for facial massage blends. Good for the more mature, dry, sensitive or inflamed skin. A source of vitamins and minerals, apricot kernel oil is excellent for restoring a glow to devitalised complexions. Has a useful element of vitamin A if not over-refined. An expensive oil to use on its own, so blend with almond, grapeseed or jojoba oils.

Avocado Oil

This oil is the most easily absorbed into the deeper levels of the skin. One of the heaviest oils, it is useful for treating mature skins. Excellent for facial massage blends as it plumps up prematurely lined skin. Contains protein, vitamins, lecithin and essential fatty acids. Useful for relieving the dryness and itch of eczema and psoriasis. An expensive oil to use on its own, so blend with other nourishing oils such as almond.

Borage Oil

Very rich in gamma linolenic acid, vitamins and minerals, borage oil is a useful addition to oils to treat skin disorders such as eczema and psoriasis. Because of its fatty acid content it is also useful as an anti-ageing treatment. Far too expensive to use neat, the easiest way to use borage oil is to pierce a capsule and add the contents to your blend.

Carrot Oil

This carrier oil is produced by a process of maceration and is a good source of vitamins (especially beta carotene) and minerals. Used to help heal scar tissue, it is useful for facial blends to combat acne and irritated skin. Apply sparingly as it will stain the skin yellow if used in excess.

Evening Primrose Oil

A rich source of gamma linolenic acid, vitamins and minerals. Excellent for face and body massage blends, especially to combat dry, devitalised skin and eczema. Again, expensive to use on its own so add the contents of one or two capsules to your massage blend.

Grapeseed Oil

A favourite with aromatherapists for its light texture and lack of smell. Grapeseed oil is non-greasy and excellent for body massage blends. Suits all skin types. It is impossible to buy completely unrefined grapeseed oil, so it needs other unrefined oils added to it to boost its lack of nutrients.

Hazelnut Oil

This oil is slightly astringent, so suits oily or combination skins. Hazelnut oil is also more easily absorbed than most so is excellent for face and body massage blends. However, it is one of the more expensive oils so dilute with grapeseed or sunflower oil.

Jojoba Oil

Jojoba oil is a wonderfully light carrier oil and the best base for facial oil blends. Because of its fine texture it is the most suitable oil for oily, combination and acned skins. Jojoba penetrates the skin more easily than most oils and is also good for body massage. Rich in vitamin E, jojoba has a longer shelf life than many other vegetable oils.

Olive Oil

This oil is easily available in its cold-pressed, unrefined state. However, it does have a slightly sticky texture so suits dryer skins. Excellent for adding to body massage blends and for soothing sore, chapped skin.

Passionflower Oil

A useful source of essential fatty acids, vitamin E and minerals. Passionflower oil helps maintain skin elasticity and is an excellent addition to face and body massage blends. The easiest and cheapest way to use it is to pierce a capsule and squeeze the contents into the mixture.

Peachnut Oil

A useful source of essential fatty acids, vitamins and minerals, peachnut oil is a very good addition to face and body massage blends. Helps prevent skin dehydration and is especially suitable for the more sensitive complexions. Has a useful element of vitamin A if not over-refined and can be used instead of apricot kernel oil

Safflower Oil

Another favourite with aromatherapists for body massage because of its light texture and penetrative power. Unrefined versions contain useful amounts of vitamins and minerals. Safflower oil is also one of the cheapest and most readily available oils.

Sesame Oil

Unrefined sesame oil contains vitamins, minerals and lecithin and is excellent for adding to facial massage blends. Can be used to help skin complaints, but the toasted variety is too pungent to use on the skin.

Sunflower Oil

A source of vitamins and minerals, this light-textured oil is especially good for body massage. Sunflower oil is also inexpensive and can be blended with the more exotic oils. Most sunflower oils are highly processed so make sure you only use the unrefined varieties that still retain their nutrients.

Wheatgerm Oil

This dark, aromatic oil is too sticky to use on its own but makes a wonderful addition to dry skin massage blends. A rich source of vitamin E so especially good for healing scar tissue and burns. Add a few drops to every massage blend as it is a natural antioxidant and will preserve the potency of all oils.

Having chosen your carrier oils, the next step is to select which essential oils to add. Essential oils are highly concentrated so should be used sparingly. As a rough guide, you need approximately 1 drop of essential oil for every 5 ml of carrier oil. Once blended, the massage mixture should be stored in a cool, dark place. A friendly chemist will sell you the small amber glass bottles that they use for medicines, and these make the best containers. Some even come with their own rubber pipettes which are useful for accurately measuring small quantities of oil.

Bath Oils

Adding essential oils to a bath is one of the easiest methods of absorbing them through the skin – and their wonderful smells turn bathtime into a whole new sensory experience!

Essential oils are destroyed by heat, so make sure the bathwater is warm, not hot. The oils should be added after the bath has run, then dim the lights, step in, relax and enjoy. As a general rule, 3–6 drops of essential oil should be sufficient. Children love fragrant baths too, and this is an easy way of using essential oils on their delicate skins without fear of irritation. Babies also have a keen sense of smell and appreciate aromatherapy treatments. Just one drop of essential oil is all that is needed for a baby bath.

Burning Oils

Essential oils were the world's first air fresheners and they are certainly more ecologically sound than chemical-laden aerosols. Oil burners are now widely available and most health food shops stock the type that are heated with night light candles. The top half of these burners is filled with water to which a few drops of essential oil are added. The drawback to this type of oil burner is that they can get extremely hot and the water quickly evaporates, leaving behind a blackened residue of burnt oil. Also, I am uneasy about leaving a naked flame unattended at any time. Electric oil burners are a high-tech solution and consist of a smooth ceramic surface which heats up at the flick of a switch. The essential oils are dropped on to its surface and kept at a constant warm temperature which is just hot enough to release the vapour without risk of burning. Safe, simple and clean, electric oil burners are ideal for offices and children's bedrooms.

Other modern methods of burning oils include fragrance rings. These are ceramic or cardboard discs that balance over the top of a light bulb. The essential oils are dropped on to the ring and the warmth from the bulb releases their aromatic odour. Do not be tempted to drop essential oils directly onto the lightbulb as this can smash the bulb. Burning essential oils is a useful way to fragrance the atmosphere. But as creative aromatherapist and cosmetics designer Jan Kusmirek points out, heating an essential oil radically alters its chemical structure. To retain the therapeutic properties of an essential oil, it is necessary to use a cold dispersal method. Glass diffusers are the best way of releasing oils into the atmosphere in their whole state. These consist of a small electric air-pump connected to an intricate series of glass tubes. When filled with neat essential oils, the pump blows air through the oil and the effect is like a mini-waterfall dispersing tiny droplets of fragrant oil into the atmosphere. A glass diffuser should be used for about 20 minutes every few hours, and some models are capable of dispersing oil into quite large areas such as hospital wards. Glass diffusers are used therapeutically in hospices and some cancer patients have found the aroma of citrus oils beneficial as they remove the depressing institutional smell.

Inhaling Oils

The rejuvenating power that essential oils possess is easily demonstrated by inhaling them. Just a few drops of eucalyptus oil sprinkled on to a tissue will instantly clear a stuffy head, while lavender oil revives and invigorates. The easiest way to inhale oils is by sprinkling a few drops on to a tissue that can then be tucked in your breast pocket or shirt sleeve. A few drops can also be dabbed on to your pillow to induce a good night's sleep. But do not use them directly on clothes as they will stain wool and other delicate fabrics. Additional methods of inhalation include adding a few drops of essential oil to a basin of hot water, covering your head with a towel and breathing the vapour in deeply. This is particularly effective for clearing a chesty cold as the hot steam helps ease congestion.

Compress Oils

The French are fond of using compresses to treat numerous skin complaints and some of the best results are seen on conditions that involve bruises and swelling. To make a compress you will need an absorbent material such as cotton wool, lint, kitchen paper or a flannel. This is then dipped into a small bowl of warm water that contains about 10–20 drops of an essential oil. Next, wring the material out so that it is damp but not dripping and apply it to the affected area. To prevent the essential oil from evaporating, wrap cling film around the entire area and cover with a warm towel. Ideally the compress should be left in place for at least an hour.

Neat Oils

Although essential oils are usually diluted or there are a few occasions that merit using them directly on the skin. Neat lavender oil is wonderfully soothing on burns, and I keep a bottle in the kitchen for this very purpose. Lavender oil also reduces subsequent burn scarring and can dramatically speed up the healing process. All essential oils are antiseptic and have many applications in first aid. Just one drop on the skin will take the initial sting out of insect bites and nettle rash.

Internal Use

Essential oils are too dangerous to be taken internally without a thorough knowledge of the subject. Some aromatherapists do prescribe the internal use of diluted essential oils for a very few, specific disorders. These are usually taken in the form of one or two drops in a glassful of water. Essential oils should only be used in extremely small quantities and, given the potentially toxic nature of some oils, it is important to be guided by a qualified practitioner. Essential oils are used as flavourings by the food and drink industry, but in relatively small amounts. Earl Grey tea, for example, is simply China tea flavoured with a few drops of bergamot oil. This oil gives the tea its pungent taste and was named after the Englishman Earl Grey who remarked on its unusual flavour while visiting a Chinese mandarin in the 19th century. Some aromatherapists advocate using other highly aromatic oils such as jasmine and peppermint to flavour tea, but this should only be done under guidance.

Properties of Essential Oils

Basil (Ocimum basilicim)

Source: Leaves and flowering tops from the herb. Native to Europe.

History: From the Greek *basileus*, meaning king. Basil is one of our oldest herbs and has been cultivated in Europe since the 12th century. Traditionally revered in India, where it is regarded as a sacred plant and dedicated to the Hindu gods Krishna and Vishnu.

Actions: Antiseptic, stimulating.

Properties: A natural tranquilliser with a mentally stimulating effect. Can help the body cope under stressful conditions. Fights fatigue but an excess can act as a depressant. A powerful oil that should not be used during pregnancy or on children.

Uses: The aroma is good at waking the senses. Burning a few drops while working encourages mental concentration. Use only as directed by an aromatherapist. Has a toning effect on the skin when used in massage blends and can be used to treat cellulite.

Bay (Pimenta racemosa)

Source: Leaves from the tree. Native to the West Indies.

History: Bay trees grow wild in the West Indies where their leaves are widely used in cooking. The leaves have a pungent taste and aroma and are especially useful to season fish and meat. Bay leaves are covered in tiny oil glands which release a delicious scent when pressed or shaken by the wind. This aromatic fragrance was especially popular with the Romans who gave bay leaf garlands to army and literary heroes, hence its Latin name *Laurus nobilis*. Bay leaf oil is traditionally associated with healthy hair and hair growth.

Actions: Antiseptic, uplifting.

Properties: A useful all-round tonic. Good for respiratory disorders and treating depression. Used to treat aches, sprains and rheumatism.

Uses: A few drops make a fortifying bath. Add to scalp oils to discourage hair loss and treat dandruff.

Bergamot (Citrus bergamia)

Source: Rind from the fruit. Native to Italy.
History: This delicately scented oil is named after the town of Bergamo in northern Italy, where it was originally cultivated. The fruit resembles a small orange and has featured in Italian herbal medicine for centuries. The oil is pressed from the oil-bearing glands on the fruit's surface, and has a deliciously fresh aroma. Bergamot oil is used to flavour Earl Grey tea and is a traditional ingredient in eau de cologne.
Actions: Antiseptic, anti-viral, uplifting, refreshing.
Properties: Useful for treating infected skin conditions such as boils, spots and acne. Aromatherapists use bergamot oil to treat infections of the urinary tract, and it can help with cystitis and urethritis.
Uses: Add to massage blends for beating depression. Bergamot has an attractive aroma that can improve mood and help focus the mind. Good for burning and adding to a relaxing end-of-day bath. Suits combination and oily skin types.

Cajuput (Melaleuca minor)

Source: Leaves and twigs from the tree. Native to Indonesia.
History: Also called the swamp tea tree, this Indonesian tree has small fragrant white flowers that cluster around a long spike. The oil is extremely aromatic and smells similar to rosemary. Traditionally mixed with olive and almond oils to soothe sunburn.
Actions: Antiseptic, uplifting, restoratives.
Properties: Improves mood, increases resistance to infections, especially coughs, colds and flu. Used by aromatherapists to treat gynaecological problems including painful periods and cystitis.
Uses: A good un-winding bath oil. Makes a highly aromatic and purifying room fragrance. Add to massage blends for its lovely fragrance and uplifting effect.

Cardamon (Ellettaria cardamomum)

Source: Seeds from the plant. Native to India.

History: Used in Eastern herbal medicine for over 3000 years, cardamon was used by the Ancient Greeks and Egyptians as incense and perfume. Hippocrates wrote that cardamon was useful for massage, and the physician Dioscorides prescribed crushed cardamon seeds for abdominal pains and fluid retention. Cardamon belongs to the same botannical family as ginger, and is used in similar ways for its warming actions.

Actions: Antiseptic, refreshing, invigorating.

Properties: A good digestive aid used by aromatherapists to treat food poisoning, nausea, heatburn and painful bouts of wind. Has a stimulating effect on the body and is used in India as an aphrodisiac.

Uses: A strongly scented oil so use sparingly. Useful to add to a warm bath to refresh and stimulate the system. All spice oils should be used with care as they can easily upset sensitive skins. Avoid during pregnancy.

Cedarwood (Cedrus atlantica)

Source: Wood shavings from the tree. Native to America.

History: Cedarwood oil is distilled from sawdust and wood shavings saved from American cedar mills. It has a distinctive aroma and was burnt in Ancient Egyptian and Greek temples as incense. The temple of Solomon in Jerusalem, commissioned by David, was built entirely of cedarwood. The amount used was so great that the forests of Lebanon have never fully recovered. Today cedarwood oil is used in many fine fragrances and aftershaves. Wood chippings from the cedar tree burnt on the fire is a subtle way of scenting a room.

Actions: Antiseptic, diuretic.

Properties: Used to treat respiratory disorders including bronchitis and catarrh. Can relieve aching muscles and help firm the skin.

Uses: Has a toning effect on the skin and can be used in oils to combat cellulite. Suits oily and combination skins and may be added to jojoba oil to treat acne.

Chamomile (Athemia nobilis)

Source: Dried flowers from the herb. Native to Europe.

History: Chamomile is named after the Greek for 'ground apple' after the apple-like scent it releases when trodden on. The lawns at Buckingham Palace are laid with chamomile and it is traditionally associated with the nobility. In Elizabethan times, dried chamomile flowers were sewn into small muslin bags and used to fragrance their once-yearly bath water.

Actions: Antibiotic, antiseptic, anti-inflammatory, calming, soothing.

Properties: A gentle, versatile oil that belongs in the first aid box. Can be used to treat nerves, headaches, insomnia, menstrual disorders and skin complaints. Especially recommended for children. Good for regulating digestive disorders, eg chamomile tea.

Uses: Wonderful in a child's bath to encourage a good night's sleep. Add to facial massage oils to soothe dry, oily or irritated skin conditions. One of the few essential oils that can be used on inflamed skin conditions.

Citronella (Cymbopogon nardus)

Source: The whole plant. Native to Africa.

History: Also known as lemon grass, this African plant thrives on dry, stony soil and also grows well in the Middle East. It has an unusually sharp, citrus smell and Alexander the Great is reported to have been invigorated by its scent whilst riding his elephant through Egypt in 332 BC. Nowadays citronella is widely used in perfume and soap-making as well as for fragrancing household cleaning products.

Actions: Antiseptic, stimulating.

Properties: Citronella is used in tropical countries as a powerful natural deodorizer. Not commonly used in aromatherapy but it is reputed to boost the immune system and can stimulate a sluggish circulation.

Uses: A few drops in a massage blend will ward off mosquitos. If you have been bitten, a small amount can be used neat on stings. May also be used neat to heal minor skin abrasions. An invigorating and refreshing oil for burning.

Clary sage (Salvia sclarea)

Source: Flowering tops and leaves from the herb. Native to Spain.

History: One of the many varieties of sage, clary sage is regarded as less toxic than the common herb. Clary sage is an attractive plant with large purple flowers and pineapple-scented leaves that carry the essential oil. Traditionally associated with feminine sexuality and gynaecology, clary sage also has euphoric properties and can induce a light-headed feeling.

Actions: Antiseptic, balancing, sedating.

Properties: Contains a hormone-like compound similar to oestrogen that regulates hormonal imbalance. Excellent to treat Pre-Menstrual Syndrome and symptoms of the menopause. Also used in abdominal and back compresses during labour to help regulate contractions. Inhaling the oil or using a few drops in the bath can lift post-natal depression.

Uses: Add to facial massage oils to treat problem skins. Excellent for massage blends applied prior to menstruation. Can be burned as a room essence to improve mood and mental clarity. Avoid during pregnancy.

Coriander (Coriandrum sativum)

Source: Seeds of the fruit. Native to India.

History: Coriander seeds are a well-known Eastern flavouring and have been used in herbal medicine for thousands of years. Coriander seeds were found buried beside Ancient Egyptians in their tombs. The name coriander comes from the Greek word *koris*, meaning bug. This is reputedly due to the fact that coriander leaves give off a pungent odour when crushed which reminded the Greeks of squashed bed bugs! Coriander has *digestif* properties and was included in the original monks' recipes for Chartreuse and Benedictine liqueurs.

Actions: Antiseptic, calming, analgesic.

Properties: Coriander is a member of same Umbelliferae family as fennel, and has similar properties. It is used by aromatherapists to treat digestive disorders and may help stimulate the appetite. The essential oil has local pain-killing properties and can help ease muscular and rheumatic pains.

Uses: Coriander is a powerful spice oil and should be used sparingly. It is useful when combined with other oils for a relaxing bath and has sedative properties. Avoid during pregnancy.

Cypress (Cypressus semperuirena)

Source: Leaves and twigs from the tree. Native to Europe.

History: This large evergreen tree is common in southern Europe. The essential oil has a similar smell and properties to pine oil. The first recorded use of cypress oil was about 2000 years ago, when Dioscorides claimed it to be a cure for diarrhoea.

Actions: Antiseptic, tonifying, diuretic.

Properties: Used to increase the circulation and as a gentle treatment for water retention. Can help improve the condition of cellulite. Useful for menopausal problems, stress and nervous tension.

Uses: Good as a burning essence for invalids. Can be added to body massage blends to improve skin tone and encourage the elimination of toxins. Has a mildly astringent action so better for oily and combination skin types.

Eucalyptus (Eucalyptus smithii)

Source: Leaves and twigs from the tree. Native to Australia.

History: Native to Australia where it is the favourite food of the koala. A pungent oil with a powerful aroma, eucalyptus oil is now principally produced for the pharmaceutical industry.

Actions: Antibiotic, antiseptic, anti-inflammatory, cleansing.

Properties: Helps clear the respiratory tract. Useful for treating sinusitis and head colds. May help relieve migraine. Use in massage oils to help ease rheumatism and arthritis.

Uses: A good burning essence. Useful as a room freshener to ease stuffiness in children and adults. A few drops in a bowl of hot water make an invigorating steam inhalation. One drop in jojoba oil is a useful treatment for acne and spotty complexions.

Fennel (Foeniculum vulgare)

Source: Seeds from the herb. Native to Europe.

History: Crushed fennel seeds are reputed to decrease the appetite and were munched by Roman soldiers on long foot marches. The seeds were also eaten by the less devout on fast days to ward off hunger pangs. Fennel is a useful diuretic and fennel tea is a helpful slimming aid as it dulls the appetite and can help reduce water retention.

Actions: Antiseptic, diuretic.

Properties: Traditionally associated with the female reproductive organs, fennel is like clary sage in that it contains a hormone-like compound similar to oestrogen. It is used by aromatherapists to regulate the menstrual cycle and can help with PMS. Fennel also helps tone and firm breast tissue, and is especially useful for promoting milk-production in women who are breast-feeding.

Uses: Although fennel is useful in baths and massage blends for toning slackened skin tissues, there are sweeter-smelling oils to choose from and it is rarely used in home treatments. The exception is breast-care and it is a key ingredient in breast massage oils for promoting lactation. Fennel should be used sparingly as an excess may induce epilepsy in prone individuals. Avoid during pregnancy.

Frankincense (Boswellia carterii)

Source: A gummy resin from the bark of the tree. Native to Somalia.

History: All parts of this tree are highly aromatic but it is the resin that is used to make the essential oil. The name comes from the mediaeval French meaning 'real incense'. Frankincense was one of the gifts brought by the Magi to the infant Christ, and has been a symbol of divinity for thousands of years.

Actions: Antiseptic, purifying.

Properties: Its unusual pungent smell helps focus the mind and this oil has meditative qualities. Used to treat stress and nervous tension.

Uses: A good oil to burn when overworked or trying to cope under pressure. A few drops rubbed into the scalp helps clear the mind and encourage mental stimulation. Suits oilier complexions but is also used in facial oils to deter fine lines and wrinkles.

Geranium (Pelargonium graveolens)

Source: The whole plant. Native to the island of Réunion.
History: There are over 700 different types of geranium flower, but only seven are used to make essential oils. The strongest scented is called Geranium Bourbon and comes from Réunion Island in the Indian Ocean. This is an important ingredient in Estée Lauder's best-selling Youth Dew perfume. Geranium oil has a rose-like aroma which comes from an alcohol called geranoil contained in the plant's leaves. Geranoil is most highly concentrated in the Rose Geranium variety. One of the most useful oils, it is traditionally associated with female sexuality and is safe for diluted external use during pregnancy.
Actions: Antiseptic, toning, strengthening.
Properties: A versatile oil used to soothe skin irritations and heal burns and minor skin abrasions. Suits all skin types and is particularly useful for treating eczema and psoriasis. Used by aromatherapists for a wide range of ailments including hormonal and menstrual problems.
Uses: Can be added to massage oil for its skin-soothing properties and wonderful floral smell. Suits all skin types including dry, oily and sensitive.

Ginger (Zingiber officinale)

Source: Roots from the plant. Native to China.
History: An important element in traditional Chinese medicine, ginger arrived in Europe via the Spice Route during the Middle Ages. Ginger is used to fight colds and infections, and the Chinese use it to treat any condition relating to an imbalance of moisture such as catarrh or diarrhoea. The essential oil has a fresh, herby smell and not the pungent aroma traditionally associated with the root. Ginger has a reputation as an aphrodisiac, and the women of Senegal still weave ginger roots into their clothing to attract the opposite sex.
Actions: Antiseptic, warming, fortifying.
Properties: Used in massage blends to treat muscular

stiffness and rheumatism. Also used by aromatherapists to treat nervous tension and anxiety. Ginger tea treats all types of nausea, especially travel sickness and morning sickness. Uses: A powerful spice oil, so use sparingly. Useful when combined with citrus oils for a stimulating bath blend. A few drops in hot water make a useful foot bath to treat colds and flu. Not suitable for highly sensitive skins. Avoid during pregnancy.

Hyssop (Hyssopus officinalis)

Source: Leaves from the herb. Native to Europe.
History: This flowering herb produces a highly fragrant oil that is an important ingredient for perfume-making. Although hyssop is native to the South of France it is also widely cultivated in Brazil and the Middle East.
Actions: Antibiotic, antiseptic.
Properties: Used to treat respiratory infections including coughs, colds and flu. Promotes the healing of bruised skin and is useful in combating the aches of rheumatism and arthritis.
Uses: A powerful oil so use sparingly and not at all during pregnancy. Use in compresses on bruised or aching limbs. Add to facial massage blends to treat dry and sensitive complexions. Hyssop gives off a warm, vibrant aroma when burned as a room fragrance.

Jasmine (Jasminum officinale)

Source: Flowers. Native to southern France.
History: Jasmine oil is one of the most expensive essential oils. The oil is extracted from palest pink jasmine flowers and develops into a rich shade of ruby red. It is an important oil for the perfume industry and is the heart of many fine fragrances, including Chanel No 5, Femme by Rochas, Samsara by Guerlain and Anaïs Anaïs by Cacharel. The highest quality jasmine oil comes from Grasse in the South of France, where it has been grown for hundreds of years. However, its production is under threat by property developers building holiday homes on many of the oldest jasmine fields. As there is no satisfactory synthetic equivalent to jasmine oil, top perfume houses

such as Rochas have had to buy their own jasmine fields to ensure sufficient supplies for their fragrances. Jasmine oil is a reputed anti-depressant and is used in Chinese herbal medicine as a general tonic.

Actions: Antiseptic, energising, uplifting, restorative.

Properties: Will invigorate and lift depression. Used to treat menstrual disorders, stress and general anxiety. In addition to its exquisitely heady fragrance, jasmine is extremely good for soothing dry, sensitive skins.

Uses: An expensive oil but it only needs to be used in tiny quantities. A few drops make a luxurious bath oil. An excellent addition to massage oils for the face and body. Reputed to repair skin tissues and can be used in small quantities during pregnancy to help prevent stretch marks. Suits all skin types, especially the sensitive.

Juniper berry (Juniperus communis)

Source: Dried berries. Native to Europe.

History: The oil comes from the ripe, dried juniper berries that grow in many regions around the world. Native to northern Europe, Juniper is an increasingly important crop in northern Asia and North Africa. Juniper berries have a pungent, aromatic smell and are used to give gin its distinctive, bitter flavour.

Actions: Antiseptic, anti-fungal, stimulating and diuretic.

Properties: A medicinal oil that is used by aromatherapists to treat digestive, urinary and hormonal problems. Also used to treat liver problems and combat chronic obesity. Reputed to strengthen the immune system.

Uses: Add a few drops to a bath to relieve tired, aching limbs. Suits oily and combination complexions. Good for treating problem skins and a few drops can be used in facial oils for treating acne. Avoid during pregnancy.

Lavender (Lavendula officinalis)

Source: Flower spikes from the herb. Native to England.

History: From the Latin *lavare* meaning 'to bathe', lavender oil is one of the most versatile of all essential oils. The oil is contained in the tiny green pods that sit either side of its pale purple flowers. Used in fragrances and skincare for centuries, lavender oil was the first English essential oil to be distilled commercially in the late 17th century. The oil is the main ingredient in lavender water which was created at about the same time. Lavender oil remains an important component of many fine fragrances.

Actions: Antiseptic, antibiotic, anti-viral, anti-fungal, balancing, fortifying, toning.

Properties: The most useful of all essential oils and a must for the first aid box. Excellent for treating infections and inflammatory disorders. Its gentle balancing action can either calm or stimulate according to what the body needs. Highly effective for treating burns. Also used by aromatherapists to treat abrasions, coughs, colds, flu, stress, nausea, ulcers, acne, boils, asthma and rheumatism. Can help relieve headaches and migraine.

Uses: Use neat to heal burns and dilute with wheatgerm oil to repair scar tissue. Add a few drops to the bath for a general fortifying effect. Can be burned in hospitals or sick rooms to promote an atmosphere of well-being. Suits most skin types except the very dry. An excellent oil for massage blends.

Lemon (Citrus limonum)

Source: Rind from the fruit. Native to South-East Asia.

History: One of the easiest oils to extract from the oil glands on the fruit's outer peel, lemon oil is a traditional antiseptic and purifier. Associated with the hair and scalp, it is reputed to stimulate hair growth and will bleach hair blonde if applied and exposed to the sun. Citrus oils should be used within a year of purchase.

Actions: Antiseptic, antibiotic, anti-fungal, diuretic, stimulating.

Properties: Used to strengthen the immune system and ward off infections. Useful to treat colds, sinusitis and sore throats. Is also used by aromatherapists to treat digestive disorders, gallstones, fever and anxiety.

Uses: Add to massage oils to help improve blood circulation and skin tone. Can be used neat in small quantities as an antiseptic. Useful for treating blemished skin. Add to massage blends to tone flabby skin and help combat cellulite. Citrus oils react strongly to sunlight and should

Do not USE MARJORAM OIL

not be used on the skin while sunbathing or before using a sunbed.

Mandarin (Citrus nobilis)

Source: Rind from the fruit. Native to Italy.
History: Extracted from the tiny glands on the rind of mandarins, this fruit is an important crop in Italy, Brazil, Spain, Argentina and China. An inexpensive oil, it is an important ingredient in cheaper fragrances. Citrus essential oils should be used within a year of purchase.
Actions: Antiseptic, fortifying.
Properties: Used medicinally as a general tonic and natural tranquilliser. Can help with insomnia, stress and nervous tension.
Uses: Add to a warm bath for an uplifting, toning effect. Use in pregnancy massage oils to boost the circulation and discourage water retention. Good for combination and problem skins. Mandarin is a citrus oil which reacts strongly to sunlight. Do not use on the skin while sunbathing or before using a sunbed.

Marjoram (Origanum majorana)

Source: Flowering tops and leaves from the herb. Native to Hungary.
History: Also known as sweet marjoram, this versatile European herb produces a spicy oil which has a warming action. In hot climates, the plant secretes a sweet, sticky resin from its stems which is popular with honey bees.
Actions: Antiseptic, calming, sedating.
Properties: Used to regulate the nervous system and treat insomnia. Induces drowsiness and an excess can have a mildly narcotic effect. Used by aromatherapists to treat menstrual problems, menopausal disorders, anxiety and stress. Can help ease aches, sprains and intestinal cramps.
Uses: Use a few drops in the bath before bedtime to promote sleep. Add to massage oils to treat strained muscles and tired, aching limbs. Suits oily and combination complexions. Avoid during pregnancy.

Melissa (Melissa officinalis)

Source: Leaves from the herb. Native to Europe.

History: Also known as lemon balm as the leaves release a lemon-like fragrance when pressed between the palms. Melissa thrives in Mediterranean countries and produces a highly fragrant oil that is popular for perfume-making. Together with angelica extract, melissa was a key ingredient in balm water made by Carmelite monks in mediaeval times. This highly prized fragrance was the world's first unisex scent and was worn by both noblemen and women.

Actions: Antiseptic, sedative.

Properties: Can help treat nerves, over-exertion and stress. Useful against digestive disorders and bacterial infections.

Uses: Use in the bath to unwind and promote relaxation. Can be added to massage blends for use after exercise. Also used to treat eczema. Suits all skin types.

Myrrh (Commiphora myrrha)

Source: Bark and resin from the bush. Native to Somalia.

History: First extracted more than 3000 years ago, myrrh comes from a small thorny bush. Originally used by the Egyptians to embalm mummies and perfume linen. Egyptian women wore small pieces of cloth impregnated with myrrh oil around their necks and its fragrance was released by their body heat. The essential oil was one of the Magis' gifts to the infant Christ. Traditionally associated with the mouth, some 2000 years ago the physician Dioscorides stated that 'myrrh doth strengthen the teeth and ye gummes'. Pliny also recorded that the ingredients for an Ancient Greek sore skin ointment called *susinum* consisted of cinnamon, saffron and myrrh.

Actions: Antiseptic, anti-inflammatory.

Properties: Useful for treating chronic chest complaints such as bronchitis and catarrh. Helps heal burns and minor skin abrasions. Improves digestive disorders and is used in the treatment of fungal infections, including candidiasis.

Uses: Popular in skincare oils to soothe angry, inflamed skin. Add a few drops to face and body massage oils to strengthen and tone the skin. Suits combination complexions and problem skins. Avoid during pregnancy.

Neroli (Citrus aurantium)

Source: Flowers from the tree. Native to southern Europe.
History: Also known as orange blossom or orange flower oil. Neroli is named after Flavio Orsini, Prince of Nerola in the 16th century, whose second wife loved the flower's fragrance. Neroli oil has a distinctively soft, fruity aroma and remains an important ingredient in modern Eau de Colognes.
Actions: Antiseptic, antibiotic, uplifting.
Properties: Warms and relaxes the body. Useful for relieving anxiety and nervous tension. Calms pre-exam or interview nerves and is used to treat stage fright. Useful for menopausal and hormonal disorders.
Uses: A few drops in a massage oil can help improve a sluggish circulation and tired complexion. Useful for blends to treat problem skins and acne. Suits oilier skin types. Creates a deliciously fragrant and fortifying bath.

Patchouli (Pogostemon patchouli)

Source: Dried leaves from the herb. Native to China.
History: The patchouli plant looks similar to lemon balm and the highly scented oil glands are scattered over its leaves. A rich, claret-coloured oil with legendary skincare attributes. Originally used in the Far East and India as an aphrodisiac and household purifier. The first recorded use of patchouli oil in Europe was by the weavers of Paisley in Scotland who discovered that they could not compete with the Indian shawl exporters unless they impregnated their cloth with the same patchouli fragrance. The essential oil has a typically heavy, Eastern aroma and is an important ingredient in many spice-based perfumes.
Actions: Antiseptic, antibiotic, anti-fungal, fortifying.
Properties: A useful, multi-purpose oil. Used to calm fevers and inflamed skin conditions. Can help treat fungal infections, acne and scalp disorders including dryness and dandruff.
Uses: A useful addition to skincare oils as it suits most complexions. Can be diluted with wheatgerm oil and used on scar tissue and burns. Good for treating problem skin conditions such as acne. Useful for toning the skin and fighting cellulite. Add to scalp oils to stimulate healthy hair

growth. Gives off an attractive, heady aroma when burned and a few drops turn bathtime into a sensual treat.

Peppermint (Mentha piperata)

Source: The whole plant. Native to Europe.
History: This pungent, fresh-smelling oil comes from the European herb named by the British botanist John Rea in 1700 for its peppery smell. Peppermint leaves contain the compound menthol which contributes to its strong smell and feeling of coldness when rubbed on the skin. Traditionally used in aftershaves and skin tonics for its invigorating action. Peppermint is also a well-known aid to digestion, eg peppermint tea. The essential oil available to the consumer tends not to keep for more than a year.
Actions: Antiseptic, invigorating, stimulating, refreshing.
Properties: Used to treat headaches, migraine and insomnia. Clears the head and encourages positive thinking. Has an anti-spasmodic action useful for relieving wind, heartburn, indigestion, nausea and colic.
Uses: Add to massage oils for its invigorating and refreshing effect. Not the best bath oil as it can make the water feel cold against the skin. Suits oily and combination complexions.

Petitgrain (Citrus aurantium)

Source: Leaves and twigs from the tree. Native to southern Europe.
History: This woody-smelling oil comes from the orange tree, traditionally grown in the warm, humid climates of southern France, Morocco and West Africa. The name petitgrain comes from the French for 'little bit', referring to the tiny droplets of oil encapsulated in the leaves.
Actions: Antiseptic, calming, fortifying.
Properties: Used to treat an overburdened nervous system. Helps relieve anxiety and tension. Useful for insomnia and as a general aid to convalescence.
Uses: Add a few drops to a bath before bedtime to promote sleep. Gives off a warm, subtle aroma when burned. Suits dry, mature and sensitive skins. An excellent oil to add to massage blends.

Pine (Pinus palustris)

Source: Needles and twigs from the tree. Native to America.

History: One of the first essential oils documented by Dr Jean Valnet for its power to prevent respiratory disorders. Pine oil is associated with cleanliness and freshness and is commonly added to medicated soaps and household cleaners.

Actions: Antiseptic, antibiotic, stimulating.

Properties: Useful for treating colds, flu, bronchitis and other respiratory infections. Strongly antiseptic, so useful for general infections and minor skin abrasions. Used by aromatherapists to help with bladder and kidney disorders and to improve the circulation.

Uses: Pine is a potent oil and should be used sparingly. Use a few drops in a bowl of hot water as a steam inhalation. Can be burned to give off a cleansing aroma. One or two drops in the bath will help stave off infections and boost a sluggish circulation. Avoid during pregnancy.

Rose Otto (Rosa damascena)

Source: Flower petals. Native to Bulgaria.

History: Also known as rose Bulgar or attar of roses, this fragrant oil comes from ruby-red damascena roses. Legend has it that the damask rose was created from a single drop of sweat falling from Mohammed's brow. The flower later gave its name to the city of Damascus and the heavy silk fabric that was originally woven there. The essential oil is now principally cultivated in the valley of Kazenlik in Bulgaria. As the sun rises over the Balkan foothills the precious oil content of the roses drops dramatically due to evaporation. The blooms that have flowered must therefore be picked very early in the morning. Genuine rose otto is distinguished by its greenish colour and at low temperatures has a semi-solid, almost crystalline texture. Pure rose oil contains over 500 different chemical constituents and so far has proved impossible for the cosmetic chemists to copy exactly. It remains one of the most important perfume ingredients and rose otto is found in many fine fragrances including Chanel No 5, Estée Lauder's White Linen and

Fidji by Guy Laroche. Rose oil is one of nature's most versatile extracts and is reported to have a specific healing action on the liver.

Actions: Antiseptic, uplifting, nourishing, soothing.

Properties: Traditionally associated with soothing dry, mature skins. Useful to treat mild depression and fatigue. Can help PMS and symptoms of the menopause.

Uses: A luxury oil to be used sparingly in facial massage blends or added in tiny quantities to a bath. A wonderful oil for children and fabulous for pampering the body during pregnancy. Suits dry, mature and sensitive skins.

Rose Absolute (Rosa centifolia)

Source: Flower petals. Native to South-East Asia.

History: Although rose absolute is widely used in aromatherapy, it is not a true essential oil. Rose absolute is produced by solvent extraction from the pale pink centifolia rose. This species bears few oil-producing glands, and is used more for its odour than any other therapeutic purpose. Following solvent extraction, rose absolute is distilled with alcohol and there is a feeling amongst many professionals that traces of the chemical solvent may be carried through to the end product. Pure rose absolute is highly concentrated and expensive. As a result, what is most commonly sold as rose essential oil is more likely to be a dilution of the absolute. Rose absolute is a very important element in perfume and the centifolia roses have been cultivated by perfumiers in Grasse since the 16th century. Rose absolute was first distilled in Persia and remains an important Middle Eastern flavouring. It is most commonly used in sweetmeats such as Turkish delight.

Action: Antiseptic, uplifting fragrance.

Properties: The main benefits from rose absolute come from its lovely smell and antiseptic properties. Although it is used in skincare, some aromatherapists feel that it may not provide the same level of nourishment offered by rose otto.

Uses: As a cheaper alternative to rose otto.

Rosemary (Rosmarinus officinalis)

Source: Flowering tops from the herb. Native to Spain.
History: One of the oldest essential oils, it is stored in tiny oil glands just beneath the leaf's surface. The aroma is easily released when the leaves are rubbed between the fingers. Regarded as a sacred herb by the Ancient Greeks and Romans, and often used in their rituals. Traditionally associated with the head, the 17th-century English herbalist Culpeper used two or three drops on the temples to relieve headaches. Rosemary oil was also the base for the world's first commercially produced perfume called Hungary water formulated in 1370.
Actions: Stimulating, antiseptic, invigorating, diuretic.
Properties: An excellent all-round tonic. Helps combat water retention and cellulite. Useful for healing sprains and aching limbs. Used to relieve headaches, dandruff and combat hair loss. Has pain-relieving properties and may help rheumatism and arthritis.
Uses: Use sparingly in massage oils or add a few drops to the bath as a pick-me-up. Can be used to tone flabby skin and help get rid of cellulite. Suits problem skins and oilier complexions. An excess can induce epilepsy in predisposed persons. Avoid during pregnancy.

Rosewood (Aniba rosaeodora)

Source: Wood chips from the tree. Native to Brazil.
History: Also known as Bois de Rose. Produced from the bark of the South American *Aniba rosaeodora* tree, so named for its lightly rose-scented wood. Used as a cheaper alternative to the genuine rose petal oils, but has far fewer therapeutic benefits.
Actions: Antiseptic, antibacterial, toning.
Properties: Used to relieve headaches and may help migraine. A good anti-depressant and useful tonic to improve mood and ward off general malaise.
Uses: An inexpensive oil which can be used in place of real rose oil for its smell, although its skincare properties are greatly reduced. Useful in body massage blends and in the bath as a pick-me-up.

Sage (Salvia officinalis)

Source: Flowering tops from the herb. Native to Europe.
History: A sacred herb from the Ancient world, sage has a distinct and strongly pungent aroma. Sage has many medicinal properties and is thought that it takes its botannical name from the Latin *salvia*, meaning salvation. Sage will grow in most parts of Britain, although our supplies of the oil tend to come from Mediterranean countries. Sage is also an important ingredient in Chinese herbal medicine.
Actions: Antiseptic, anti-fungal, stimulating, healing, toning.
Properties: A useful regulator of the central nervous system. Aromatherapists may use sage to treat depression, severe menstrual and digestive disorders. Useful against catarrh, bronchitis and other chest conditions.
Uses: A powerful oil which can overstimulate. Use only under the guidance of an aromatherapist and not at all during pregnancy.

Sandalwood (Santalum album)

Source: Sawdust and wood chippings from the tree. Native to India.
History: A traditional Indian extract, this oil comes from a parasitic tree that grows by attaching its roots to others. It has a rich, woody aroma and is burned by Hindus in temples and at all their religious occasions. Hindu spiritual leaders paint their foreheads with sandalwood paste as a symbol of purity. Sandalwood comes from one of the slowest growing trees and it takes 40 years before the essential oil can be extracted from its bark. The wood itself is popular for furniture-making as it resists attack from pests, notably woodworm.
Actions: Antiseptic, comforting, a reputed aphrodisiac.
Properties: Sandalwood oil has a high natural alcohol content so it is strongly antiseptic. A versatile and gentle oil that provokes calm and a sense of well-being. Can also help with Pre-Menstrual Syndrome and is reputed to strengthen the immune system. Used by aromatherapists to treat impotence.

Uses: Use a few drops in the bath as a pick-me-up. Can be added to massage blends to treat sore, inflamed skin conditions. Suits irritated, flaky complexions and is useful in facial oil blends for blemishes and acne.

Tea Tree (Melaleuca alternifolia)

Source: Leaves and twigs from the tree. Native to Australia.
History: This interesting oil comes from the bark of a common Australian tree which is extremely resistant to disease. The tea tree also has amazing powers of recuperation and if chopped down will quickly grow again from its original stump. The essential oil is highly renowned for its anti-viral and anti-fungal properties. Originally used in aboriginal medicine, tea tree oil is being increasingly used by conventional medics to treat skin disorders and fungal infections including candidiasis (thrush) and ringworm. Tea tree oil is five times more effective for killing germs than household disinfectant and at the same time is far kinder to the skin.
Actions: Antiseptic, antibiotic, anti-viral, anti-fungal.
Properties: Very useful against fungal and bacterial infections. Can help ward off coughs, colds and flu. Used to treat skin disorders including cold sores, warts and burns. Trials by Australian dermatologists have shown tea tree oil to be as effective at treating acne as orthodox treatment using benzoyl peroxide, but with far fewer side-effects.
Uses: Use neat in very small amounts to treat spots, burns and insect bites. Add to scalp oils to treat dandruff and scalp disorders. A few drops in the bath can combat the effects of shock and hysteria.

Thyme (Thymus vulgaris)

Source: Flowering tops from the herb. Native to Europe.
History: A medicinal herb known to the Ancient world that is now used in herbal medicine throughout the world. Commonly burnt as a household disinfectant to ward off rodents and get rid of fleas. Sprigs of fresh thyme can be hung in wardrobes instead of moth-balls. Thymol is the principal active constituent in this oil and as it is a powerful antiseptic it must be used with caution.

Actions: Antiseptic, antibiotic, anti-fungal, anti-viral, sti-muulating.
Properties: Used by aromatherapists as a general tonic to relieve fatigue and anxiety. Stimulates the circulation and encourages the elimination of toxins. Reputed to strengthen the immune system. Useful for tired, aching limbs. Can help regulate the menstrual cycle and lower blood pressure.
Uses: A powerful oil that should be used under the guidance of an aromatherapist and not at all during pregnancy.

Vetiver (Vetiveria zizanoides)

Source: Dried roots from the grass. Native to India.
History: Although native to India, this wild grass is now grown in many volcanic areas as its extensive network of roots helps to protect the soil. The essential oil has a fresh 'green' fragrance and is used in many perfumes and aftershaves.
Actions: Antiseptic, calming, soothing.
Properties: This sweet-smelling oil is used by aromatherapists to lower blood pressure, reduce nervous tension and promote relaxation. Used in massage as a muscle relaxant.
Uses: Use a few drops in the bath before bedtime to relax and induce sleep. Add to massage blends to reduce redness and inflammation. Suits problem skins and oily complexions.

Ylang Ylang (Cananga odorata)

Source: Flower petals. Native to Indonesia.
History: An attractive, flowering tree originally grown in Indonesia but now cultivated in the Comoro Islands, northwest of Madagascar. Its flowers are bright yellow and have long flowing petals. The name ylang ylang comes from the Malay for 'flower of flowers'. The essential oil smells similar to jasmine and was an original ingredient in the famous Macassar oil. Today, ylang ylang is a key ingredient in the Estée Lauder perfume Beautiful.
Actions: Antiseptic, invigorating, a reputed aphrodisiac.
Properties: Regulates the nervous system and lowers blood

pressure. Useful during times of depression, stress and overwork. Used as a general tonic but an excess can cause headaches. Some aromatherapists use ylang ylang as a treatment for impotence and frigidity.

Uses: Use with caution in massage blends as it can occasionally provoke an allergic reaction. Add a few drops to a warm bath to revive the body at the end of a long day. When burned the fragrant aroma helps combat anxiety and depression. Suits normal and combination skin types.

Golden Rules

To preserve the potency of an essential oil blend it is important to store it in the right conditions. All oils should be kept in metal or amber glass bottles to protect them from spoilage from the light. Essential oils should not be stored in plastic containers as they can dissolve chemicals within the plastic which ruin the purity of the oil. Essential oils must always be tightly sealed, preferably with a screw-top lid and not a cork. Oils are affected by the air each time they are opened so buy in small quantities and always replace the lids. Oils last longer if kept in a cool place, such as in a box at the top of the fridge. If this is not possible, make sure the room temperature where they are kept does not exceed 15° C (59° F)

Words of Caution

While most essential oils have many health and beauty benefits, some are unsafe for home use and should only be used under the guidance of a qualified aromatherapist. These include clove, cinnamon, sage, thyme and wintergreen. Essential oils should also be used with great care during pregnancy as they have been shown to enter the bloodstream and may cross the placental barrier. It is impossible to be sure of the effect, if any, that essential oils might have on a developing baby. In addition to those oils already mentioned, the following must be avoided during pregnancy: basil, hyssop, marjoram, myrrh and rosemary, and all spice oils such as ginger and coriander. Essential oils can be very useful during pregnancy though, and the safest oils for the expectant mum are chamomile, geranium, sandalwood and very diluted citrus oils. Rose may also be used after the first trimester. To be on the safe side, I recommend consulting an aromatherapist before using any essential oils during pregnancy, especially during the early stages. If you are already pregnant, or suspect you might be pregnant, it is important to tell your aromatherapist before beginning any treatment. Essential oils are largely safe to use in skincare blends, but some of us do have more sensitive skins than others and even quite common ingredients can cause allergic reactions. This is also true of essential oils, and those more likely to irritate the sensitive include basil, lemon grass, rosemary and ylang ylang.

For some less reputable companies, the term 'aromatherapy' has become a licence to print money. Poor quality oils are certainly cheaper to produce but have far fewer therapeutic properties. However, it is hard for us to tell exactly what is in the bottle and so we must rely largely on the integrity of the producers. As a general guide, you mostly get what you pay for and the more expensive oils are usually worth the extra cost. Many high street aromatherapy ranges count on pretty floral packaging instead of high grade ingredients and for this reason I prefer to buy my oils by mail order from specialists accredited by the International Federation of Aromatherapists (address at the end of this book). If you do buy oils over the counter, always read the label first. Those called 'fragrance oils', 'aromatic oils' or 'aromatherapy oils' are not essential oils at all, but inferior dilutions. They may contain all kinds of unwanted extras including synthetic perfumes and preservatives.

Pure essential oils are powerful substances and must be treated with respect. They should be kept well out of the reach of children, not left lying around for small, inquisitive hands to open. If an essential oil is accidentally swallowed, drink as much water as possible and seek immediate medical attention. Essential oils will cause pain and irritation if splashed in the eyes. If this happens, flush with plenty of water and consult your doctor if the pain does not subside. Don't forget that all essential oils are also highly flammable.

7

Health and Beauty Remedies

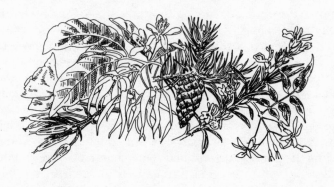

Pure plant oils are the most valuable and versatile ingredients for natural health and beauty remedies. They are also a wonderful way of caring for the skin. I base my entire skincare regime on oils and firmly believe them to be the best extracts for nourishing the skin, preventing spots and warding off wrinkles. Plant oils are not only useful for creating a clearer complexion, they make good treatments for the rest of the body too. The skin secretes its own natural oil (sebum) through sebaceous glands all over the body. Sebum is designed to keep our skins smooth and if we don't produce enough of it our skin quickly becomes rough, dry and devitalised. Our sebum levels are influenced by many factors, including diet, lifestyle and hormonal changes, and any slight imbalance can easily lead to skin problems. The best way to restore our own natural oil levels is by using pure plant oils. These are far more compatible with our own natural body oil than many synthetic skincare ingredients commonly used today.

Pure plant oils can be used in many ways to maintain

the body beautiful. Apricot and peach kernel oils restore suppleness and elasticity to even quite mature complexions, while jojoba oil is good for problem skins and acne. The action of these oils is further enhanced by adding essential oils according to your own requirements. Our skin is constantly on the move, shedding dead cells and facing different elements with each change of season. The beauty of using blended oils on the skin is that the formulas can be continually adjusted to reassess your skincare needs. Another significant factor is that plant oils are also the cheapest form of skincare. Although some of the remedies given in this chapter include the more exotic oils, most are based on everyday ingredients that can be found in every supermarket. Even the more expensive essential oils and cold-pressed nut oils will save you money in the long run. Instead of spending vast sums on separate moisturisers, skin tonics, face masks, perfumes and body treatments, all you really need are a few well-chosen oils.

As we have seen, many natural oils have powerful healing properties and can help with severe skin conditions such as acne and eczema. We can obtain their benefits in several different ways including bath oils and fragrant massage blends. In addition to their many therapeutic properties, plant oils also leave the skin wonderfully smooth and deliciously scented. And it is not only the skin that benefits from the application of plant oils, they are also very useful for encouraging stronger nails and improving the strength and condition of our hair. The plant oil remedies detailed in this chapter are designed to be used in conjunction with the *Vital Oils Beauty Diet*. If you decide not to follow the diet, you should boost your essential fatty acid and vitamin intake with a beauty oil supplement such as evening primrose, borage, almond, peachnut, passionflower or avocado.

Oils for the Face

Moisturisers

Oils for the face serve several important functions. Most importantly, they can be used as moisturisers to lubricate and soften the skin, leaving it smoother and more elastic.

Avocado and hazelnut oils have richer textures than most and are excellent as night-time treatments or for nourishing very dry skins. These two oils also appear to have the greatest penetrative powers and are able to slip through the uppermost layers of skin cells to feed the fresh, young cells forming underneath. By supplying the skin with high levels of essential fatty acids, plant oils are able to strengthen the fragile cellular membranes and act as natural anti-agers. Many unrefined oils also contain useful amounts of vitamin E which fights free-radical cell damage, the principal cause of premature ageing. Because dryness is determined by water loss and not the amount of sebum produced, even oily skins can become dehydrated and flaky. Jojoba oil is the best choice to moisturise combination and oily skin types as it has the lightest texture and won't clog the pores or encourage blackheads. Plant oils can be used as a moisturising base under make-up, but allow the oils a little time to sink in before applying foundation. You may find that you don't need to use the oil all over the face, but just over the drier cheek and eye areas. As most remedies call for only a few drops of the essential oils it may be cheaper to ask a local aromatherapist to make them up for you – although some shops do now offer facilities to blend your own oils instead of having to buy a full bottle of each ingredient. Jojoba oil is naturally long-lasting and most of the other oil blends contain a few drops of wheatgerm oil to act as a natural preservative. However, don't make up more than you need and always store your supplies in a cool, dark place.

Facial oils are a highly emollient alternative to moisturising creams and lotions. They are quick and easy to make – simply shake the oils together and store in an amber glass bottle. Facial oils are also highly economical to use as they should be applied sparingly. Three or four drops are all you need to treat the entire face and neck.

Normalising Facial Oil
25 ml (1 fl oz) jojoba oil
25 ml (1 fl oz) peachnut or apricot kernel oil
5 drops wheatgerm oil
10 drops lavender, 5 drops geranium, 5 drops neroli essential oils

Dry Skin Facial Oil
25 ml (1 fl oz) avocado oil
25 ml (1 fl oz) peachnut or apricot kernel oil
Contents of 5 passionflower oil capsules
10 drops wheatgerm oil
10 drops sandalwood, 5 drops geranium, 5 drops rose essential oils

Combination Skin Facial Oil
50 ml (2 fl oz) jojoba oil
10 drops lavender, 10 drops geranium essential oils

Oily Skin Facial Oil
This blend contains citrus oil so avoid sunbathing after applying.
50 ml (2 fl oz) jojoba oil
10 drops patchouli, 5 drops lemon, 5 drops cypress essential oils

Anti-Ageing Facial Oil
This blend makes an excellent night-time treatment and is a good alternative to expensive skin-serums.
25 ml (1 fl oz) almond oil
25 ml (1 fl oz) jojoba oil
Contents of 5 evening primrose oil capsules
10 drops wheatgerm oil
10 drops frankincense, 10 drops geranium essential oils

Devitalised Skin Facial Oil
A good tonic for tired, stressed skins.
25 ml (1 fl oz) jojoba oil
25 ml (1 fl oz) peachnut or apricot kernel oil
10 drops wheatgerm oil
5 drops lavender, 5 drops neroli, 5 drops jasmine essential oils

To Help Eczema
Apply sparingly on inflamed areas.
50 ml (2 fl oz) peachnut or apricot kernel oil
Contents of 10 evening primrose oil capsules
10 drops wheatgerm oil
5 drops chamomile essential oil

To Help Acne
Apply sparingly each morning to thoroughly cleansed skin.
50 ml (2 fl oz) jojoba oil
10 drops cypress, 5 drops tea tree, 5 drops patchouli
essential oils

Facial Massage

One of the most effective ways to use oils on the face is in
conjunction with a simple facial massage. The best time to
do this is in the evening before bed when you are at your
most relaxed. There are several beauty benefits to be gained
from gently massaging the face. Firstly, it will stimulate
fresh blood supplies and increase the levels of oxygen
within the skin. Secondly, localised massage will boost the
lymphatic system responsible for clearing waste matter
from skin cells. The lymphatic system is a much underrated
and important part of the body. It consists of a network of
lymph channels which run parallel to blood vessels
throughout the body. These channels are filled with a pale,
milky substance called lymph which acts as the body's
dustman. Lymph's main function is to carry away the
toxins and decomposed cellular material that have a nasty
habit of clogging up the system. Unlike our blood supply,
however, lymph doesn't have a heart to pump it around
the body, and relies on external exercise and movement to
stimulate its flow. By using a specific series of 'lymphatic
drainage' massage techniques, we can encourage the
speedy elimination of toxins that lead to a clearer, healthier
complexion. With a bit of practice, the facial massage
techniques don't take more than a couple of minutes, and
it is well worth getting into the habit of using this routine
every night.

Facial Work-Out
The Warm Up   Pour a little of your chosen face oil on to
the fingertips and smooth over a thoroughly cleansed face
and neck. Using the fingertips, lightly tap the skin all over,
starting at the hairline and working down across the face
and throat. Repeat the tapping movements, this time
beginning from the base of the throat and moving
upwards. Using the tip of the middle finger on each hand,

lightly smooth the skin across the forehead, cheeks and chin. Use the backs of the fingers to smooth the skin under the chin in soft outward movements.

Lymph Drainage   With the middle fingertip of each hand, gently press along each eyebrow and around the entire eyesocket. Next, place both fingertips beside the corner of the inner eye and smooth the skin downwards following the line under each cheekbone. This sweeping movement should finish beside the earlobes. Finally, use the thumbs and index fingers to gently pinch along the jawline, starting at the chin and working out towards the ears.

Face Pullers   These facial exercises help tone and strengthen the underlying connective tissues that support the skin. They may look a little strange to anyone watching, but will bring fresh oxygen supplies to the surface of the skin and kick-start the lymphatic system into action. Begin by opening the eyes as wide as you can and lifting the brows upwards in a surprised expression. Holding this position, try to close your eyelids. You will feel the muscles of the entire eye, forehead and temple areas start to work. Repeat five times. To exercise the cheeks, mouth and jawline, exaggerate saying the words 'week' and 'queue'. Repeat 20 times, making the mouth stretch as far as it can with each word. The final exercise is for firming up the saggy skin under the chin that can lead to jowls and a double chin. Start by sticking your neck out, then bring the bottom lip over the top lip, and hold for five seconds. You should feel a significant pull on these rarely used muscle groups in the upper neck. Repeat five times.

Cleansers

The idea that oils can act as cleansers as well as moisturisers may sound surprising, but they are highly effective at drawing out dirt and embedded grime. Oil cleansers work on the proven principle that oil dissolves best in oil, not soap and water. The hot oil cleansing method given below is especially good for removing excessive sebum and all oil-based make-up. The lighter plant oils, such as jojoba, can be used neat to remove eye make-up and will shift even the most stubborn waterproof mascara. All oils should be used sparingly around the eye area, however, as an excess may leave a greasy film across the eye and could clog the tear ducts.

Pour a little of the hot oil cleanser into one hand and warm by rubbing the palms together. Smooth over the entire face and neck and lightly massage into the skin with small, circular movements. The heat comes from a soft flannel or face cloth wrung out in hand-hot water. Gently wipe away all traces of the oil with the flannel, rinsing at least twice in more hot water. Use the cloth to gently buff away dead skin cells, concentrating on the chin, nose and nostrils to discourage blackheads. When all the oil has been removed, wring the flannel out in cold water and dab over the skin to tighten and tone the tissues. Wash the flannel regularly to keep it fresh and germ-free.

Hot Oil Cleanser for Normal Skins
50 ml (2 fl oz) jojoba oil
50 ml (2 fl oz) almond oil
10 drops lavender essential oil

Hot Oil Cleanser for Dry Skins
50 ml (2 fl oz) almond oil
50 ml (2 fl oz) avocado oil
10 drops rose or sandalwood essential oils

Hot Oil Cleanser for Combination/Oily Skins
100 ml (4 fl oz) jojoba oil
10 drops bergamot or mandarin essential oil

Flower waters

These flower waters make wonderfully refreshing skin tonics and can be used on cotton wool to wake the face up first thing in the morning. Wipe over the face after cleansing, taking care to avoid the immediate eye area. Flower waters are also useful stored in a water-spray and lightly spritzed over foundation to set it in place. Flower waters are made with water and essential oils and are the perfect alternative to commercial skin tonics containing alcohol, synthetic fragrance and preservatives, all of which are potentially irritating. Do not use plain tap water as this contains a cocktail of chemicals including chlorine, nitrates, fluoride and aluminium, none of which has any place in skincare. The best water to use is either filtered tap water or still mineral water with a low sodium and nitrate content. Flower waters are made by pouring all the liquids together into a bottle or jar and shaking vigorously before each application. They have a limited shelf life and should be made in small amounts and used within a few weeks. Keep your floral waters cool – the fridge is the perfect place for storing sprays to freshen the face during the summer.

Normalising Flower Water
100 ml (4 fl oz) water
5 drops lavender, 5 drops neroli essential oils

Dry Skin Flower Water
100 ml (4 fl oz) water
5 drops sandalwood, 5 drops rose essential oils

Combination/Oily Skin Flower Water
100 ml (4 fl oz) water
5 drops lavender, 5 drops lemon essential oils

Instantly Reviving Flower Water
100 ml (4 fl oz) water
5 drops neroli, 5 drops peppermint essential oils

Skin Scrubs

The fastest way to brighten dull, dingy-looking skin is with a natural face scrub. These contain finely ground particles designed to buff off dead skin cells that give the complexion a grey or sallow appearance. By sloughing away the uppermost layer of dead skin cells we can also speed up the rate of cell renewal. This means that fresh young cells from the deeper levels of the dermis reach the surface of the skin more quickly. Encouraging cell renewal helps to ensure a healthy turnover of cells within the skin, and will delay many of the more visible signs of ageing. The best way to use a skin scrub is to dampen the face with a little warm water and rub the scrub into the skin with the fingertips. Dead skin cells don't take much dislodging, so don't over-scrub as this could damage delicate capillaries on the cheeks and stimulate the sebaceous glands into producing excessive sebum.

Dry/Sensitive Skin Scrub
½ a ripe avocado
15 ml (1 level tbsp) fine ground oatmeal
5 ml (1 tsp) almond or olive oil
The oil released by the avocado when rubbed over the skin is supplemented with a small amount of additional plant oil. Use once or twice a week to gently lift dry flakes of skin, leaving the complexion soft and smooth.

Combination/Oily Skin Scrub
7.5 ml (½ level tbsp) ground almonds
25 ml (1 ½ level tbsp) medium ground oatmeal
5 ml (1 tsp) fresh lemon juice
water to mix
This mixture will help deep cleanse the skin and discourage spots and blackheads. Use three times a week, but take care not to rub too hard and over-excite the sebaceous glands.

Beauty Boosters

Our skin is constantly exposed to the harshness of the elements, environmental pollution and the dehydrating effects of central heating and air conditioning. Regular face masks and herbal steams are the easiest and most effective way to repair the damage and encourage a glowing complexion. These oil-based skincare remedies are designed as instant facial pick-me-ups and are the perfect way to prepare for a special night out or simply to use as a skin-pampering treat.

Normal/Dry Skin Treatments

Moisture Mask
½ a ripe avocado
5 ml (1 tsp) honey
1 egg yolk

The perfect treatment for dry, more mature skins. Mix all the ingredients together and apply to a thoroughly clean face and throat. Relax for 15 minutes while the skin absorbs the nutrients from this nourishing mixture. Avocados have the highest oil and protein content of any fruit and also contain useful amounts of vitamins A, B complex, C and E, iron and potassium. Egg yolk is our richest source of lecithin which has the ability to lock moisture into the skin.

Avocado Revitaliser
Ripe avocado skin
1 avocado stone
½ a ripe avocado
15 ml (1 tbsp) plain live yogurt
5 drops jasmine essential oil (optional)
This skin treatment is in three stages and uses every single part of the oil-enriched avocado. Begin by rubbing the inside of the avocado skin over a thoroughly cleansed face and neck. This has a naturally exfoliating action and is a good way of gently dislodging dead, dingy skin cells. The inside of the avocado skin is also a good source of oil and contains a humectant capable of holding moisture in the skin. The next stage of the treatment is to roll the avocado stone gently over the face and neck using the palm of your hand. This increases blood circulation and boosts the lymphatic system. It also triggers the multitude of pressure-points that improve the skin's appearance. Finally, mix the remaining face mask ingredients together and smooth over the face and neck. Leave on for at least 10 minutes before rinsing away with warm water. Follow with a few drops of face oil for devitalised skins.

Mature Skin Treatments

Facial Firmer
30 ml (2 level tbsp) linseed
60 ml (4 tbsp) hot water
3 drops petitgrain essential oil
rectangular muslin cloth or cotton gauze
This unusual facial compress contains cracked linseed, which has the extraordinary ability to draw out excess fluids from puffy skin and firm sagging skin tissues. Place

the linseed in a grinder and whizz for a few seconds to split the seeds. Mix the seeds with the hot water and essential oil until they form a sticky paste. Spread the mixture over one half of the fine cotton muslin or gauze, folding the other half over the top to seal the compress. Place the hot linseed compress over the lower half of the face and neck, or the forehead and leave for 10 minutes. The compress can also be covered with a warm towel to retain the maximum amount of heat. The mixture may also be applied straight from the bowl, but I find it too slippery to stay put. Hot linseed compresses work well on specific areas of the face, such as a double chin, and should be used twice a week for a month to see maximum benefit.

Fragile Skin Refiner
30 ml (2 level tbsp) fine ground oatmeal
15 ml (1 level tbsp) wheatgerm
½ a ripe avocado
Dampen the oatmeal and wheatgerm with a little water before stirring in the mashed or finely sieved avocado. Mix to a smooth paste. Gently rub half the mixture over dampened skin to dislodge dead skin cells and rinse with warm water. Then smooth the rest of the mixture over the entire face and throat and leave for 15 minutes before rinsing again. This treatment works by gently lifting the dead cells that dull the complexion and immediately feeding the fresh skin cells beneath with the oil-enriched avocado and wheatgerm.

Tired Eye Compress
30 ml (2 tbsp) jojoba oil
15 ml (1 tbsp) witch hazel
2 drops chamomile essential oil
Combine the ingredients together in a glass bottle or jar and leave in the fridge to cool. Shake well before applying to cotton wool pads. Place over the eyes and relax for 20 minutes. The witch hazel and chamomile will help reduce puffiness and inflammation and the jojoba oil will nourish the fragile skin tissues around the eye area and discourage crow's feet. A very useful treatment for eyes strained by spending lengthy periods staring at a VDU or computer screen.

Combination/Oily Skin Treatments

Deep Cleaner
15 ml (1 level tbsp) fuller's earth
15 ml (1 tbsp) water
15 ml (1 tbsp) fresh lemon juice
5 drops lavender essential oil
Excellent for problem skins and treating teenage acne. Fuller's earth is a natural powdered clay and easily available in small packets from the chemist. It is very good at drawing out impurities from the skin and tightening surface tissues. Mix all the ingredients together to form a smooth paste. Leave on the face until the mixture dries before rinsing off with warm water. Wipe the face with cotton wool soaked in floral water for combination/oily skins. This removes any remaining traces of the mask and will tone and freshen the complexion.

Bacteria Buster
30 ml (2 tbsp) freshly chopped pineapple
15 ml (1 tbsp) plain live yogurt
5 ml (1 tsp) runny honey
5 drops tea tree essential oil (optional)
This face mask sorts out spotty, acne-prone skin and is a useful monthly treatment to keep the skin clear. Fresh pineapple contains the enzyme bromalin which digests the spot-forming bacteria that live on the skin and helps keep the face spot-free. The live yogurt provides beneficial bacteria to fight local infection, and the honey is included as a natural antiseptic. Tea tree essential oil is a useful addition when treating severe spots and acne. Mix all the ingredients together in a food processor. Leave on the skin for 20 minutes before rinsing with tepid water.

Spot Zapper
5 ml (1 tsp) jojoba oil
1 hot flannel
cotton buds
lavender or tea tree essential oil
This is a foolproof way to get rid of blackheads and other minor skin blemishes. Begin by adding a few drops of lavender or tea tree oil to a basin of very hot water. Hold

the head over the water and let the vapour gently open the pores. Placing a towel over the head and shoulders will ensure that the steam does not escape. With scrupulously clean fingertips, lightly massage the jojoba oil over the face. Wring the flannel out in hand-hot water and hold against the areas to be treated (avoiding the eyes). This further softens the skin and helps draw out any deeply embedded waste-matter. Blackheads are then ready to be gently squeezed, but may need several treatments before they're drawn out completely. Don't be too zealous – most spots respond better to several gentle attemps at removal instead of one vigorous one. Apply a dab of neat lavender or tea tree oil to heal every spot treated, using a fresh cotton bud each time to prevent cross-infection.

Fast Facial Steams

When time is tight and you need an instant beauty booster, nothing works more quickly than a fast facial steam. Simply add the drops of essential oil to a basin filled with hot water, cover your head with a towel and let the fragrant vapour cleanse the pores and stimulate the circulation. Those with sensitive skins or tiny broken capillaries should use steams with care, as prolonged use can aggravate these conditions. Facial steams should be followed with a cool, refreshing spray of flower water.

For Normal Skins
3 drops lavender, 3 drops mandarin essential oils

For Dry Skins
3 drops rose, 3 drops chamomile essential oils

For Combination Skins
3 drops lavender, 3 drops cypress essential oils

For Oily Skins
3 drops lemon, 3 drops eucalyptus essential oils

Oils for the Body

Skin scrubs should not stop at the neck as they are an excellent way of improving all-over skin tone. Common problems of pimply upper arms and 'chicken skin' thighs can be swiftly solved with an oil-based skin scrub. These scrubs are best used before stepping into the shower and work by sloughing off the dead skin cells and boosting the blood and lymphatic circulations. By whisking away the uppermost skin cells, the surface of the skin becomes more receptive to any body oil applied immediately afterwards. These oils are then able to penetrate more deeply and will have a more profound effect on the body.

Soft Skin Salt Rub
45 ml (3 level tbsp) fine sea salt
1 very ripe avocado
3 drops lemon essential oil
Mix all the ingredients together in a bowl before rubbing handfuls vigorously over the body. The sea salt is gently exfoliating and has a cleansing action on the skin, while the oil-enriched avocado pulp counteracts any dryness from the salt. Follow with the after-bath massage oil.

Dry Skin Body Scrub
30 ml (2 level tbsp) medium ground oatmeal
30 ml (2 level tbsp) ground almonds
1 egg
2 capsules evening primrose oil
Mix the ingredients together to form a rich paste. Rub gently over the entire body, concentrating on the upper arms, elbows, knees and thighs. Follow with the dry skin body oil.

Spotty Skin Body Scrub
30 ml (2 tbsp) finely ground aduki beans or lentils
15 ml (1 level tbsp) medium ground oatmeal
15 ml (1 tbsp) grapeseed oil
6 drops lemon essential oil
Dampen the skin and rub the mixture across the shoulders and lower back. Get your partner to scrub the bits you can't reach! Follow with the spotty back massage oil.

Anti-Cellulite Thigh Scrub
30 ml (2 tbsp) finely ground aduki beans or lentils
15 ml (1 level tbsp) coarsely ground oatmeal
15 ml (1 tbsp) grapeseed oil
30 ml (2 tbsp) witch hazel
6 drops juniper or cypress essential oil
This treatment may seem more than a little masochistic, but it certainly gets the circulation going. Blend the ingredients together to form a thick paste. Using the palms of the hands, firmly massage the mixture across the thighs, hips and buttocks. Rub the surface of the skin with circular movements, massaging the entire area for at least three minutes before showering off with alternate blasts of cool and icy water. Follow with the anti-cellulite massage oil.

Oils for Bathing

Nothing is more luxurious than sinking into a wonderfully fragrant and relaxing bath at the end of a long, hard day. Oils can be used in several different ways for bathing and are one of the easiest and most effective all-over beauty treatments. The simplest method is to add a few drops of essential oils to a pre-run bath. As essential oils are broken down by heat they should be added at the last moment just before stepping in. You can experiment with your own favourite fragrances or try these traditional bath oil blends.

The Great Unwinder
5 drops cypress, 3 drops lavender, 2 drops cajuput essential oils

All-Over Energiser
5 drops peppermint, 3 drops neroli, 2 drops jasmine essential oils

Quick Pick-Me-Up
5 drops lemon or mandarin, 5 drops ylang ylang or bergamot essential oils

Immune System Strengthener
5 drops tea tree, 3 drops lavender, 2 drops cajuput or neroli essential oils

The Aphrodisiac
5 drops patchouli, 3 drops ylang ylang, 2 drops jasmine essential oils

The Sleep Inducer
5 drops chamomile, 3 drops vetiver, 2 drops melissa essential oils

The Comforter
5 drops sandalwood, 3 drops lavender, 2 drops clary sage essential oils

Using essential oils in the bath is one of the fastest ways of getting them absorbed into the bloodstream, but they can also be used just as effectively in the shower. Mix your chosen essential oils with a little warm water and pour over a flannel or sponge. Rub the flannel or sponge vigorously all over the body just before stepping under the shower. This scented mixture can also be used while in the shower instead of synthetic perfumed shower gels. After using essential oils in the bath or shower you should gently pat the skin dry with a large, soft towel. The more relaxing oils will leave you feeling sleepy, so make sure you have time to put your feet up for half an hour afterwards.

Holistic Body Oils

Body oils are marvellous for softening and re-hydrating the skin after bathing. Soaking in the bath is great for relaxing the body but it can leave the skin slightly dry, especially on those areas of the body that contain few sebaceous glands, such as the arms and lower legs. Body oils can be used instead of body lotions to moisturise and perfume the skin. They can also have therapeutic properties according to the oils included in the blend. A weekly massage is the ideal beauty booster for the entire body. You can massage yourself, but it's more relaxing – and more fun – if you get your partner to do it for you. Begin by pouring a little oil into the hand and warming it by rubbing the palms together. Start on the soles of the feet and work up the legs with smooth, firm strokes. Concentrate on the hips and thighs to help break down any fatty deposits and discourage the formation of cellulite. Use gentle, clockwise circular motions over the stomach. This action is very soothing and helps to improve the digestion. The back is a much neglected expanse of skin and will look, and feel, much better for a rub down with body oil. You should also pay particular attention to the upper arms and elbows, often the driest areas on the body.

After-Bath Body Oil
100 ml (4 fl oz) grapeseed oil
5 ml (1 tsp) wheatgerm oil
5 drops lavender or chamomile essential oil
An excellent multi-purpose oil that has a light, non-greasy texture. Can be used sparingly in the morning after bathing as it won't leave sticky traces on clothes.

Dry Skin Body Oil
50 ml (2 fl oz) almond oil
50 ml (2 fl oz) grapeseed oil
5 ml (1 tsp) wheatgerm oil
5 ml (1 tsp) evening primrose oil
5 drops sandalwood essential oil
A nourishing oil especially useful for extra-dry skins during the menopause, pregnancy or other hormonal changes. May be used to treat eczema and is safe for most sensitive, inflamed skins. Evening primrose oil can be bought in a dropper bottle or obtained by piercing a capsule with a pin and squeezing out the contents.

Stimulating Body Oil
100 ml (4 fl oz) grapeseed oil
5 ml (1 tsp) wheatgerm oil
5 drops cajuput, 5 drops peppermint essential oils
A refreshing body oil that will wake up the senses in the morning and which has a non-sticky texture, so can be used before getting dressed. Use before exercise to warm up the muscles.

After-Sport Muscle Rub
100 ml (4 fl oz) grapeseed oil
5 ml (1 tsp) wheatgerm oil
5 drops cedarwood, 5 drops rosemary essential oils
An invigorating oil that will help ease aches and pains and prevent muscle stiffness. It has a light, spicy unisex smell.

Anti-Cellulite Oil
50 ml (2 fl oz) grapeseed oil
5 drops wheatgerm oil
5 drops juniper, 5 drops cypress, 5 drops lemon or mandarin essential oils
Cellulite is not an easy problem to treat, but using this massage blend twice a day on the affected areas will stimulate the circulation and encourage the dispersal of trapped toxins. The essential oils in this blend are powerfully diuretic and will help firm up flabby skin. Best applied after using the anti-cellulite skin scrub.

Spotty Back Massage Oil
50 ml (2 fl oz) jojoba oil
10 drops tea tree, 10 drops lavender essential oils
An excellent, lightweight oil for clearing up spots and pimples on the back and shoulders. Best applied after using the spotty back skin scrub.

After-Sun Soothing Oil
50 ml (2 fl oz) grapeseed oil
50 ml (2 fl oz) virgin olive oil
15 ml (1 tbsp) wheatgerm oil
10 drops chamomile essential oil
A suntan is simply a sign of damaged skin and is one of the main factors in skin ageing. However, you can repair some of the damage caused by the sun's rays with this nourishing oil. It has a high vitamin E content and will help minimise free-radical cell damage caused by over-exposure to the sun.

The Ultimate Relaxing Body Oil
100 ml (4 fl oz) grapeseed oil
15 ml (1 tbsp) wheatgerm oil
5 drops neroli, 5 drops sandalwood essential oils
A wonderful blend for combating the effects of stress and restoring a sense of well-being. Concentrate on massaging the knots out of the shoulders, which is where most of us hold our tension.

Earn extra Cash on a Full or Part-time
basis working from home.
Ideal for both Men and Women

No experience required
as full training will be given

A PHONE CALL **NOW** COULD MAKE
THE 1990's VERY PROSPEROUS FOR **YOU**

For details contact: HELEN

Telephone Brighouse 400516

IS

THIS

YOU?

DO YOU WANT

£10-£1,000 EXTRA P.P.WEEK

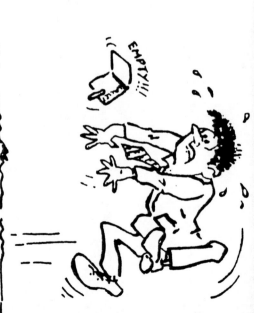

EMPTY!!!

Oils for the Hands

Our hands are the hardest working parts of our body, but also the most neglected. And if we are not careful, our hands will betray our age far faster than the lines on our face. This is because the skin on our hands ages much more quickly, and without adequate care we can end up with slack skin, deep lines and darkened areas of pigmentation known as liver spots. Our hands need constant protection from the everyday assault of harsh soaps and detergents, as well as care to combat their constant exposure to the elements. Hand models, who make their living from their hands, know the perils of the everyday tasks we take for granted, and even wear rubber gloves to wash their hair! The skin on the back of our hands has few sebaceous glands to provide natural moisture – and the skin on our palms doesn't have any at all. As a result, the hands dry out more quickly than the face and are prone to chapping in cold weather. One benefit noticed by those testing the *Vital Oils Beauty Diet* was the improvement in severely dehydrated skin conditions, including the hands feeling less chapped. While vegetable oils and oil supplements are useful to take internally for reducing skin dryness, many of the richer plant oils also make useful hand creams.

Hand Massage Oil
50 ml (2 fl oz) jojoba oil
50 ml (2 fl oz) sesame or almond oil
10 drops rose, jasmine or sandalwood essential oils
A daily hand massage helps keep the hands soft, supple and smooth, and this blend is light enough to use every day. Sesame and almond oil are a natural sunscreen and will act as a mild filter against the damaging effects of the sun that can cause liver spots. The essential oils are added mainly for fragrance but will also soothe dryer, more mature skins.

Overnight Hand Healer
½ a ripe avocado
30 ml (2 tbsp) almond oil
1 egg yolk
This is a wonderfully sticky formula for repairing severely chapped and out-of-condition hands. The oil-enriched

avocado combines beautifully with the almond oil, while the egg yolk provides protein and lecithin to lock moisture into the skin. Mix all the ingredients together to form a smooth paste. Coat each hand and slip on a pair of thin cotton gloves (from good chemists and glove departments). Leave overnight to allow the goodness from the oils to soak into the skin.

Nail growth can be an accurate reflection of inner health, and those with long, strong nails generally have a stronger physique. Nails consist of a dead protein called keratin, and begin life about 5 mm (¼ inch) below the visible lanula, or half-moon. Nails are made up of layers of keratin sandwiched together with natural oils which keep the nail flexible and strong. The nail plate is sealed to the skin by a hardened layer of cuticle which prevents dirt and bacteria from entering the finger. The appearance of our nails is due in part to the lottery of our genes and the shape and structure of nails is largely hereditary. If you compare your own hands and nails with those of your mother, you will probably see a strong resemblance. However, nail strength and their rate of growth are two factors which we can influence.

Nail growth is notoriously slow, on average about 1 mm (¹⁄₁₆ inch) a week. This means that it takes almost five months for a completely new nail to form. A well-balanced diet is vital for healthy nail growth. Nails need calcium, iron and zinc together with vitamins A, D and E. Deficiencies of these nutrients soon show up in the nails. Spoon-shaped nails may be due to anaemia (iron deficiency) and white spots on the nail are sometimes caused by a lack of zinc. Essential fatty acids are also important for maintaining the natural oils in the nail responsible for their strength and flexibility. The fact that many of those on the *Vital Oils Beauty Diet* found their nails improved is probably due to their increased intake of essential fatty acids. Again, oil supplements are a useful way of improving the state of our nails and those containing almond oil seem to be especially helpful. The speed at which nails grow not only depends on our diet, but also varies according to the season. They seem to grow faster in the summer, and more rapidly when we are young or pregnant. Finger nails grow at a much faster rate than toe nails, and this is probably due to the amount of daily exercise they receive. Typists and concert pianists have also been noted for their extremely fast-growing finger nails. A daily nail massage is a good way to encourage growth and is an excellent precautionary measure to prevent splitting and breakage.

Daily Nail Massage Oil
50 ml (2 fl oz) almond oil
10 ml (2 tsp) peachnut or apricot kernel oil
5 drops geranium or rose essential oil
This is a strengthening blend of oils designed to penetrate the cuticles and prevent them from becoming hard. Massage over the entire nail area at least once a day, concentrating on the base of the nail to stimulate healthy growth.

Problem Nail Oil
50 ml (2 fl oz) almond oil
15 drops tea tree, 10 drops bergamot essential oils
Fungal infections are common nail disorders and include paronychia (nail inflammation), onycholysis (nail separation) and onychomycosis (nail discoloration). These can be treated with a twice-daily massage with problem nail oil. Tea tree essential oil is the key ingredient in this blend as it has powerful anti-fungal properties. If symptoms persist, however, you should consult your doctor.

Hot Oil Manicure
You will need:
60 ml (4 tsp) daily nail massage oil)
nail scissors, nail file, rubber hoof stick, acetone-free nail varnish remover, cotton wool, cotton buds
Nails respond best to regular, gentle treatment, and a weekly hot oil manicure is the ideal way to keep them in good shape. Begin by removing any old nail varnish with acetone-free remover. If you find that nail varnish removers leave your nails feeling dry, add a few drops of almond oil to the bottle. Remove all traces of varnish by wiping a cotton bud soaked in nail varnish remover around the cuticles. Shorter nails are not only more fashionable now, but they are far stronger too. Trim the nails with a small

pair of scissors and file off the rough edges. Don't seesaw the nail file backwards and forwards, but file in one direction only. Never file the nails into a point as this weakens them and encourages splitting. Never cut the cuticles either as this can lead to infections. If your cuticles need attention, file away any hardened edges with a nail file. Soak the nails in the nail massage oil for at least 15 minutes, using any remaining oil to gently massage the fingers, hands and wrists. Once the cuticles have been thoroughly softened they can be gently eased back with a rubber hoof stick. This is the gentlest method of caring for the cuticles and also the most effective. The rubber hoof stick should be used moist, so dip in nail massage oil before use. Finally, if you want to re-varnish your nails, remove any greasy traces from them with cotton wool and a little nail varnish remover. Always use a clear base-coat before applying coloured varnish to prevent staining.

Oils for the Hair

The texture, shape and style of our hair can change the way we look more radically than any other aspect of our appearance. Hair is commonly described as our 'crowning glory', but for most of us it is more often a tangle of dry ends, greasiness and scalp disorders.

Oils work on the hair in two important ways. When included in our diet they nourish the hair follicles from the inside and applied directly to the hair they soften and smooth its appearance. There is far more to our hair than meets the eye and most of its development occurs underneath the skin and it is worth getting to grips with its physiology before beginning any treatment. Our body is covered with tiny hairs which sprout from follicles in the skin, these occur more densely on the scalp. The role of our hair is to prevent heat loss from the body and to provide a further layer of protection for the brain. Each strand of hair begins life about 3 mm (⅛ of an inch) below the surface of the scalp. It is made up from the same dead protein called keratin that makes our nails, and grows from a group of cells called the matrix in the hair bulb or root. Hair is produced as the living cells in the hair root die and are pushed up through the follicle. Because each strand of hair is technically dead, there is little we can do to improve its structure. Hair grows at the rate of approximately 0.35mm daily (about one hundredth of an inch) every day. As each strand grows, it pushes its way through the layers of skin, past the sebaceous glands, until it finally reaches the outside world. It then continues to be lubricated with sebum until it falls out some 2–5 years later. Hair has three distinct phases of development – a growing phase (anagenic), a resting phase (catagenic) and a falling-out phase (telogenic). When a hair reaches the end of its falling-out phase its life is over, and it is replaced by a fresh new strand.

The only way to really improve the structure of our hair is to treat it while it is still forming inside the scalp. And the most effective way to do this is by increasing the levels of certain foods in our diet, notably vegetable oils rich in vitamins and the all-important essential fatty acids.

Those who tested the *Vital Oils Beauty Diet* for even a short time noticed that their hair's condition dramatically improved, so could the foods that we eat be linked to our hair's health? The roots of our hair rely on a steady stream of nutrients to maintain healthy hair growth and any interruption to this will certainly affect our hair. Hair growth is slowed by deficiencies of vitamins A and E, two nutrients that play a large part in the *Vital Oils Beauty Diet*. In addition, most types of hair loss are governed by the male hormone testosterone. Both men and women can suffer from an imbalance of this hormone which may result in permanent hair loss. We know that essential fatty acids are vitally important for regulating the prostaglandin activity linked to hormone production. By boosting our intake of essential fatty acids it is reasonable to assume that we can help reduce hormonal related hair loss. The rate at which our hair turns grey is due to the reduced activity of an enzyme called tyrosinase. This enzyme regulates the amount of melanin produced in the hair's pigment cells that control its eventual colour. Tyrosinase activity is also related to prostaglandin production, and may also be improved by increasing our intake of essential fatty acids.

All the evidence points to an important link between the role of essential fatty acids in the diet and premature hair loss and greying, but this has yet to be proved conclusively. Meanwhile, there are many other hair and scalp disorders which we know can be improved by diet. Hair needs several specific nutrients for healthy growth, and many cases of hair loss, dandruff and weak, brittle hair stem from deficiencies in the diet. Hair roots are fed by oxygen, vitamins and minerals delivered via the blood supply. A network of arteries brings these nutrients to the hair roots, while the veins carry away the resulting waste-matter and carbon dioxide. Because the rate of hair growth is so slow, it can take 2–3 months for the effects of any dietary deficiencies to show up. Rats have a faster hair growth rate than humans, and when fed a diet deficient in essential fatty acids their fur quickly falls out and their skin becomes dry and scaly. The same is true of the human hair and scalp, only this time the effects are more gradual.

The commonest scalp disorders are dandruff and a dry, flaky scalp and both stem from problems in the production of sebum. Under-active sebaceous glands result in a dry scalp and poorly moisturised hair, while an excess of sebum can trigger dandruff. Dry scalp conditions may be due to many factors, including cheap, harsh shampoos and the over-use of a hot hair dryer. The condition is usually helped by an increase of essential fatty acids in the diet. Atopic eczema and psoriasis can also cause a flaky scalp, and may again be helped by oil supplements. The diagnosis of dandruff is notoriously difficult and only a few people with flaky scalps actually suffer from true dandruff. Dandruff is caused by micro-organisms that feed on a build-up of sebum on the scalp. This is why it is so important to wash the hair every day. There is no evidence to suggest that washing the hair every day encourages dandruff or greasy hair – in fact, the reverse is true. Provided you use a shampoo with a mild detergent base and don't rub too hard and over-stimulate the sebaceous glands, daily washing can help both these problems. Unfortunately, most cheaper shampoos contain harsh detergents that can irritate a sensitive scalp. Even baby shampoos may not suit the sensitive, as the main reason for their association with baby care is the fact that they don't sting the eyes. Dandruff is also a hormone-related problem and attacks are often triggered by stress. Again, oil-enriched foods that promote the production of prosta-glandins can be very helpful. Both dry scalp conditions and dandruff are helped by avoiding saturated and hydrogenated fats in the diet, and an increase in essential fatty acids. The essential fatty acids also strengthen the cellular membranes that hold the hair shaft together as it grows beneath the scalp, and help maintain its tensile strength and flexibility.

Our hair suffers more abuse in the name of beauty than any other part of the body. Harsh chemicals from perm solutions, peroxide and hair colourants can irretrievably damage the structure of our hair. While the over-use of hot hair driers, heated rollers, hair lacquers, gels, sprays and styling mousses leaves it dull, dry and thoroughly devitalised. The easy answer is to reduce the level of abuse we inflict on our hair. For example, try switching your hair dryer to a cooler setting or leaving it to dry naturally once in a while. But once the damage has been done the best way to restore a glossy shine is with an oil-enriched conditioner. Conditioners work by smoothing down the scales on the hair cuticle that surrounds each strand. By flattening these tiny scales, the hair reflects more light and appears shinier. It also becomes sleeker, more manageable and less likely to tangle. Oil-enriched conditioners are especially important for hair which has been chemically treated by perming or colouring. These processes tend to leave the hair shafts more porous and low in natural moisture. Hot oil treatments are especially useful for restoring bounce and shine to these devitalised hair types. However, it is of little use trying to repair split ends with any kind of conditioner. Once the hair has broken it is impossible to seal it back together again. The dry ends sealer detailed on page 170 is one of the best treatments to prevent hair from splitting, but the only real cure is to snip the ends off and start again.

Daily Hair Shiner
50 ml (2 fl oz) grapeseed oil
25 ml (1 fl oz) jojoba oil
10 drops wheatgerm oil
5 drops frankincense or sandalwood essential oils
Shake the oils in a bottle until thoroughly blended together.

Use a tiny amount every day – one or two drops is literally all you need for a glossy shine. Apply by dropping the oil on to the palm of one hand, rubbing the palms together and then smoothing through the hair ends. This oil is also good for adding texture and body to layered hair.

Dry Ends Sealer
25 ml (1½ tbsp) almond oil
25 ml (1½ tbsp) olive oil
25 ml (1½ tbsp) peachnut or apricot kernel oil
5 drops wheatgerm oil
Mix the oils together and apply to the hair ends only. This mixture has a heavy texture and is useful for temporarily sealing split ends, but is too sticky to use near the roots or scalp.

Hair Loss Hair Pack
30 ml (2 tbsp) avocado or hazelnut oil
15 ml (1 tbsp) wheatgerm oil
1 beaten egg
Blend all the ingredients together and massage into the scalp. Wrap the head in a hot towel and leave for at least an hour to allow the oils to absorb into the scalp. This hair pack is rich in vitamin E, essential fatty acids, protein and lecithin. Of course it won't restore hairs on a perfectly smooth, bald pate, but regular use can discourage hair loss by feeding the follicles with the nutrients they need for healthy growth. This hair pack is highly emollient and may need two or three gentle shampooings with warm, not hot, water to remove every last trace.

Dry Hair Mayonnaise
½ a ripe avocado
1 egg yolk
5 ml (1 tsp) fresh lemon juice
60 ml (4 tbsp) olive or sunflower oil
Beat the egg yolks in a food processor or with a wire whisk while slowly adding the oil. Stir in the finely mashed pulp of the avocado and the lemon juice. The mixture should have the consistency (and taste!) of mayonnaise. Coat the dry hair strands with the mixture, and work into the scalp. Wrap the head in a hot towel to seal in body heat and

promote greater absorption. Leave for at least half an hour before rinsing with tepid water. Use a mild shampoo to remove all remaining traces of the mixture. This hair pack is excellent for dry and chemically treated hair and should be used at least once a month. Any left-over mayonnaise may be eaten.

Scalp Massage Oil
50 ml (2 fl oz) jojoba oil
50 ml (2 fl oz) almond oil
5 drops rosemary, 5 drops bay essential oils

Another important factor in maintaining a healthy head of hair is a daily scalp massage. This brings fresh blood supplies to the hair follicles and ensures they receive a steady supply of nutrients. Scalp massage also dislodges the dead skin that accumulates around the hair roots causing itchiness and flaking. Blend the oils together and rub a few drops of the mixture over the palms and fingers before massaging the scalp with firm, kneading movements. Leave for a few minutes to soften the skin before washing the hair with a mild shampoo. This massage oil is also excellent for treating cradle cap in infants, but the rosemary essential oil should be substituted with 3 drops of chamomile. The action of the massage should also be much gentler. A twice-weekly treatment is suitable for babies of all ages and will remove the build-up of dead, flaky skin, keeping the scalp clear.

Anti-Dandruff Oil
50 ml (2 fl oz) jojoba oil
8 drops tea tree, 3 drops cedarwood, 3 drops lavender essential oils

Mix the oils together and gently massage into the affected areas. Leave overnight and shampoo as usual the following morning. Use each night for a fortnight to see maximum results. Tea tree oil is a powerful anti-fungal agent and can help with many scalp disorders. However, if symptoms persist, consult your doctor or trichologist.

Charts

Cooking Oils

Name	saturates	Fat Type mono-unsaturates (Oleic)	poly-unsaturates (Linoleic)	Culinary uses
Almond	10%	70%	20%	dressings, flavouring
Corn	12%	25%	57%	light frying, baking
Hazelnut	8%	77%	10%	dressings, flavouring
Olive	14%	70%	10%	all, including deep-frying
Safflower	10%	12%	73%	light frying, sauces
Sesame	15%	40%	40%	sauces, dressings, flavouring
Sunflower	15%	30%	50%	light frying, sauces
Walnut	10%	15%	55%	dressings, flavouring

NB The composition of all oils varies due to differences in analytical technique, growing conditions and environmental factors. Grapeseed, groundnut, rapeseed and soybean oils have not been included as they are not generally available in an unrefined state.

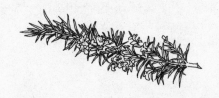

Oil Supplements

Name	Key Characteristics
Avocado	9% Linoleic acid
Borage	37% Linoleic acid, 25% GLA
Cod Liver Oil	20% long-chain Omega-3s (8% EPA, 9% DHA)
Evening Primrose Oil	70% Linoleic acid, 9% GLA
Fish Oils*	30–50% long-chain Omega-3s (15% EPA, 10% DHA)
Linseed	60% Alpha Linolenic Acid (short-chain Omega-3s), 14% Linoleic acid
Passionflower	73% Linoleic acid
Peachnut	34% Linoleic acid

*Composition of fish oil varies even more than other oils, depending on the type of fish, feeding grounds, stage of breeding cycle etc.

Essential Oils

Name	Properties
Basil	Antiseptic, mentally stimulating
Bay leaf	Antiseptic, uplifting
Cajuput	Antiseptic, uplifting, restorative
Cardamon	Antiseptic, refreshing, invigorating
Cedarwood	Antiseptic, diuretic, toning
Chamomile	Antibiotic, antiseptic, calming, soothing
Citronella	Antiseptic, stimulating, refreshing
Clary sage	Antiseptic, balancing, restorative
Coriander	Antiseptic, calming
Cypress	Antiseptic, toning, diuretic
Eucalyptus	Antibiotic, antiseptic, anti-inflammatory
Frankincense	Antiseptic, purifying, meditative
Geranium	Antiseptic, soothing, strengthening
Hyssop	Antibiotic, antiseptic, warming
Jasmine	Antiseptic, energising, uplifting, aphrodisiac

Juniper berry	Antiseptic, anti-fungal, diuretic, stimulating
Lavender	Antibiotic, antiseptic, anti-viral, anti-fungal, balancing
Lemon	Antibiotic, antiseptic, anti-fungal, diuretic, stimulating
Lemon grass	Antiseptic, toning, refreshing
Mandarin	Antiseptic, fortifying, refreshing
Marjoram	Antiseptic, calming, sedating
Melissa	Antiseptic, sedating, balancing
Myrrh	Antiseptic, anti-inflammatory, anti-fungal
Neroli	Antibiotic, antiseptic, uplifting, fortifying
Patchouli	Antibiotic, antiseptic, anti-fungal, fortifying
Peppermint	Antiseptic, invigorating, stimulating, refreshing
Petitgrain	Antiseptic, calming, fortifying
Pine	Antibiotic, antiseptic, stimulating
Rose absolute	Antiseptic, uplifting, soothing
Rosemary	Antiseptic, stimulating, diuretic
Rose otto	Antiseptic, uplifting, nourishing, soothing
Rosewood	Antiseptic, uplifting, toning
Sage	Antiseptic, anti-fungal, stimulating, fortifying
Sandalwood	Antiseptic, comforting, uplifting, aphrodisiac
Tea Tree	Antibiotic, antiseptic, anti-viral, anti-fungal, cleansing
Thyme	Antibiotic, antiseptic, anti-fungal, anti-viral, stimulating
Vetivert	Antiseptic, calming, relaxing
Ylang Ylang	Antiseptic, invigorating, aphrodisiac

Glossary of Terms

Antioxidant – A substance capable of preventing damage to cells caused by oxidation and free-radicals.

Aromatherapy – The therapeutic use of essential oils in massage.

Carrier oils – A vegetable oil base in which essential oils are dissolved.

Cholesterol – A fat-like substance produced by the liver and also found in some high-fat foods. Cholesterol surrounds every cell in the body and is needed to maintain nerve fibres, produce hormones and transport fats around the body.

DHA – Docosahexaenoic acid. A long-chain Omega-3 polyunsaturate only found in fish oils.

Enfleurage – The traditional method of extracting floral essential oils by soaking in sheets of animal fat or beeswax.

EPA – Eicosapentaenoic acid. A long-chain Omega-3 polyunsaturate only found in fish oils.

Essential fatty acids – Polyunsaturated fatty acids which are termed "essential" as they are required for good health. These cannot be synthesised by the body and must be supplied in the diet.

Essential oil – fragrant, volatile and highly concentrated essences extracted from leaves, flowers and roots of plants. In this case, the term "essential" refers only to the fact that they are essences.

Free-radical – Highly active and destructive chemical compounds from oxygen produced by oxidation.

GLA – Gamma Linolenic Acid. A fatty acid occurring naturally in breast milk, borage and evening primrose oil. Can also be produced in the body from linoleic acid.

HDL – High-Density Lipoprotein. A type of blood fat that helps to prevent cholesterol deposits from settling in the arteries.

Hormones – Substances produced by glands in the endocrine system that have an action on organs or tissues. Examples are corticosteroids from the adrenal cortex, growth hormone from the pituitary gland and oestrogen mainly from the ovaries.

Hydrogenation – The process of combining polyunsaturated oils with hydrogen to convert them into solid fat.

LDL – Low-Density Lipoprotein. A type of blood fat that carries cholesterol deposits in the bloodstream. An excess can lead to a cholesterol build-up in the arteries.

Leukotrienes – Hormone-like substances involved in inflammation in the body.

Monounsaturates – Fatty acids containing one double-bond. These are highly resistant to oxidation and are relatively stable at high temperatures. They also have a slight lowering effect on cholesterol in the bloodstream and seem to preserve the optimum HDL:LDL ratio.

Oxidation – A process whereby a substance is chemically combined with oxygen and its original structure altered or destroyed.

Polyunsaturates – Fats containing two or more double-bonds. These reduce the level of cholesterol in the bloodstream but may also adversely affect the HDL:LDL ratio.

Prostaglandins – Hormone-like substances that control biological functions in the body.

Saturated fats – Fatty acids that raise cholesterol levels, usually of animal origin and solid at room temperature, eg butter and lard. Saturated fats also block the health-giving properties of essential fatty acids.

Smoke Point – The temperature to which a cooking oil may be heated before producing smoke.

Stroke – Damage or clinical death of part of the brain due to a blockage in its blood supply.

Thrombosis – A frequently fatal condition caused by a blood clot blocking the main artery to the heart or brain.

Triglyceride – The basic structure of all oils and fats. Also a fatty component in the blood related to heart disease.

Vitamin F – An incorrect name for essential fatty acids.

Useful Addresses

Aromatherapy

The International Federation of Aromatherapists
4 Eastmearn Road, London SE21 8HA.
Send an SAE for a list of local accredited practitioners and aromatherapy training courses. They also publish a regular newsletter which gives details of suppliers of high quality essential oils.

Aromatherapy Associates
68 The Maltings, Fulmead Street, London SW6
Supply excellent ready-made massage blends, electric oil burners and provide occasional training seminars for beauty therapists.

The Association of Tisserand Aromatherapists
PO Box 746, Hove BN3 3XA
Will provide details of aromatherapy training under the direction of Robert Tisserand.

London School of Aromatherapy
PO Box 780, London NW5 1DY
Send a large SAE for details of training courses and list of their trained aromatherapists countrywide.

Health

Action for Research into Multiple Sclerosis (ARMS)
4a Chapel Hill, Stansted Mountfitchet, Essex CM24 8AG

National Eczema Society
Tavistock House North, Tavistock Square, London WC1H 9RS

The Disfigurement Guidance Centre
Guild House, 1 George Street, Cellardyke, Fife KY10 3AS

Please send an SAE when contacting any of the above organsations.

Further Reading

The Eskimo Diet by Dr Reg Saynor and Dr Frank Ryan, Ebury Press.

Fats, Nutrition and Health by Robert Erdmann Ph.D. and Meirion Jones, Thorsons.

The Food Pharmacy by Jean Carper, Simon and Schuster.

Evening Primrose Oil by Judy Graham, Thorsons.

World of Herbs by Lesley Bremness, Ebury Press.

The Practice of Aromatherapy by Dr Jean Valnet, C W Daniel Co. Ltd.

The Aromatherapy Handbook by Daniele Ryman, C W Daniel Co. Ltd.

Marguerite Maury's Guide to Aromatherapy by Marguerite Maury, C W Daniel Co. Ltd.

Aromatherapy for Everyone by Robert Tisserand, Penguin.

The Complete Book of Massage by Clare Maxwell-Hudson, Dorling-Kindersley.

General Index

Index of Recipes